FATE IS BULLSHIT

A LOGICAL GUIDE TO HAPPINESS

JOEY FRANCESS

© 2024 Joey Francess

All rights reserved. No part of this publication may be reproduced, distributed, or transmitted in any form or by any means, including photocopying, recording, or other electronic or mechanical methods, without the prior written permission of the publisher, except in the case of brief quotations embodied in critical reviews and certain other noncommercial uses permitted by copyright law.

Published by Giuseppe Sarto

ISBN: 978-1-0688767-1-4

Library and Archives Canada Cataloguing in Publication

Title: Fate is Bullshit: A Logical Path to Happiness

Names: Joey Francess

Identifiers: ISBN: 978-1-0688767-1-4

Special Thanks

This couldn't be done with out the help of my friends and family.
Specially my Mother and Father.

CONTENTS

INTRODUCTION 6

Section 1
LOGICAL HAPPINESS 9
    Freewill 10
    The Secret To Happiness 15
    Nobody's Perfect 19
    The Advice Paradox 22
    Kill Them With Kindness 25
    The Art Of Leaning In 30
    Amor Fati: Embracing Fate 33
    The Past Is A Place Of Reference, Not A Residence 37
    The Duality Of Motivation: Light And Dark Side 43

Section 2
SELF FOCUS 46
    Self-Awareness And Self-Esteem 47
    Motivation And Praise 50
    Gratitude 54
    Expectation And The Thief Of Joy 59
    What Are You Worth? 64
    Should You Lie? 68
    Fear And The Pursuit Of Acceptance 73

Section 3
HABITS 78
    Done Is Better Than Perfect 79
    Be Careful Of What You Want Because You Might Just Get It 82
    What You Want Vs What You Want To Want 87
    Rome Wasn't Built In A Day 90
    Only Dead Fish Go With The Flow 95

How Much Are You Willing To Take?.. 98
Gambling Your Future Happiness: The Sunk Cost Fallacy. 102
Walking Away 108

Section 4
LESSONS TO FOLLOW 112
Kintsugi.. 113
Social Media: The Mirror You Didn't Know You Were
Looking Into 116
100 Years In Perspective 118
Is Happiness Contagious?... 121
The Spotlight Effect 124
Do The Clothes Make The Person? Or Is It
The Person Who Makes The Clothes Look Good? 128

Section 5
PERSONAL REFLECTION... 133
You Never Learn Anything On A Good Day 134
Age Vs Experience... 138
Good Health Is Indeed A Crown On A Well Person's Head .. 143
Worrying Does Not Take Away Tomorrow's Troubles; It
Takes Away Today's Peace.. 147

Section 6
WISDOM 151
The Three-Second Rule.. 152
The Power Of Accommodation... 157
The Oxygen Mask Theory 162
Saying You Can't, Is Saying You Won't Even Try 165
The Scorpion And The Frog: A Parable Of
Nature And Trust.. 170
Confirmation Bias 175
Naive Optimism 181
Reflections On Life's Lessons 186

CONCLUSION 189

INTRODUCTION

First things first, I want to thank you for buying this book. More importantly the intention to read it. Before we get started, I want to offer a bit of a disclaimer. I want you to know that in no way am I trying to change your thoughts, ideas, and most importantly your beliefs. This book is based on my thoughts and ideas and at the very least is intended to get you thinking. Some things may seem controversial to you. Whether you agree or disagree, I hope it helps on your journey through life. A lot of people inspired me, so I hope to inspire you. Life is a journey filled with ups and downs, twists and turns, joys and sorrows.

Along the way, we encounter countless obstacles and opportunities, each presenting us with the chance to learn, grow, and evolve into the best versions of ourselves.

Yet amidst the chaos, it's easy to lose sight of our inner compass and become overwhelmed by the amount choices and challenges we face.

Using logic as a roadmap to personal growth, self-discovery, and ultimately, a more meaningful and fulfilling existence. Drawing upon psychological insights, philosophical wisdom, and real-life anecdotes, each chapter of this book serves as a catalyst, illuminating the path forward and empowering you to think outside the box and chart your own course toward happiness and success.

As you delve into the pages of this book, you'll embark on a journey filled with practical wisdom, deep insights, and actionable advice aimed at helping you unlock your full potential and craft a life that truly aligns with your innermost values and dreams. From honing your self-awareness and cultivating gratitude to facing life's trials with resilience and grace, each chapter presents a fresh perspective on the art of living well amidst life's ever-changing landscape. Together, we'll explore the concept of free will and the profound impact of our choices, unravel the mysteries of logical happiness and fulfillment, and tap into the transformative power of adopting a growth mindset. We'll delve into the importance of bouncing back from adversity, the significance of chasing meaningful goals, and the dangers of falling prey to negative thoughts and self-doubt.

But perhaps most importantly, we'll uncover the immense influence that our mindset, attitudes, and beliefs exert on how we perceive and experience the world around us.

So, whether you're seeking guidance on surmounting personal hurdles, pursuing your passions with unwavering determination, or simply craving inspiration to live your best life, "Fate is Bullshit" serves as a logical roadmap to steer you through the unique twists and turns of your own personal journey. Together, let's embark on this voyage of self-discovery, delving into the depths of the human experience and unearthing the timeless wisdom that resides within each of us. Let's confront life's obstacles head-on, armed with courage, curiosity, and an unshakeable belief in the resilience of the human spirit.

SECTION 1
LOGICAL HAPPINESS

FREEWILL

First things first, which do you believe? Do we have free will, or is everything predetermined? I've personally spent a lot of time pondering this question. Even in discussions with others, the answer is never clear. Most people think it's usually a mixture of the two. That always led me to further contemplation of one versus the other. "How could they be mixed?" I'd ask myself. The simple answer is, they can't.

Let's start with determinism. If everything is preplanned, a destiny so to speak, that means your life is your life. No matter what decision you make, you're essentially following the script that destiny has already written for you. There is no changing it, whatever it may entail. Whether it's heartache, diseases, car accidents, or war, it's all part of the predetermined course. If you ask me, that's a very hard pill to swallow. How could there be a higher power that condemns individuals in any way for no reason? If "it's meant to be" because we must learn a lesson. What would the point of the lesson be if it's all pre-written? It's not like we can learn from our mistakes and improve; that's up to destiny, which has already decided. The only valuable lesson would be to accept life however it may unfold (which is a very stoic perspective and does have its usefulness).

And just to top it off, if this is really the case, why not indulge in vices like smoking, drinking, drugs, or laziness? Whatever is coming to us is coming to us, good or bad. Destiny will provide as we have no control over our own lives. There are too many points here that, when said out loud, just sound absurd.

So, what about Free Will? I personally think the idea that we have complete control of our lives scares people. The notion that we are where we are because of all the decisions we've made makes people uneasy because they have no one else to blame but themselves. Free Will is a very simple concept: the power to make decisions or perform actions independently without the constraint of necessity or fate. Very simply put, you act at your own discretion.

Imagine you get into an argument with someone, you get so frustrated that you want to hit them (for the record, I never condone violence). You decide to knock their teeth out, and when the police arrive, you plead your case that this person made you do it. They got you so mad that you just had to shut them up. The truth is you chose to hit them; you could have walked away. They truly didn't make you do anything. You acted at your own discretion.

This is where things get interesting. I believe we are all connected, and I mean literally connected, not just in a spiritual way. Using the example I just gave, let's imagine you are the one who's annoying others. You are speaking passionately about a subject and are being genuine. You have no intention of upsetting anyone or speaking with malice. Later that day, you had an important meeting or even a date with a new fling. Yet because of your conversation (and the other guy punching you), you now have a few teeth missing. Instead of going to the meeting, you went to the hospital, once excited for your date now looking for an excuse to get out of it without hurting your ego.

The actions of one (or reaction in this case) have changed the path of your future. So, if it was destiny's plan to have you ace this meeting and get a promotion or marry this fling and start a family, those plans have now changed because of the actions of someone else. Because you didn't go on this date, your fling found someone else. Your coworker got the promotion instead of you and is now your boss, flaunting it in your face every day. Some people would say that it was just meant to be. I could say sometimes shit happens. Did you know this person was aggressive? Could you have avoided it entirely knowing it might set them off? That makes it your choice.

Everything in life is based on cause and effect. Sometimes we can predict the outcomes, and sometimes we can't. Sometimes we need to completely change our entire plan, and sometimes our plan comes together perfectly. There's a funny saying, "If you want to make God laugh, tell him your plans." The truth is your plans may fail because of the Free Will of those who are a part of it. Just because you want things to go a certain way doesn't mean everyone else agrees with you.

Just like two people going for the same job, just because you want it doesn't mean the other candidate will back out. Whether you get it or not, it's not God's or Destiny's will; it's the free will of the person making the choice to pick you or not. If you get it, you don't need to thank God, and if you don't, it doesn't necessarily mean it wasn't meant to be. It was just the choice of another person, another person acting at their own discretion.

This idea of meant to be or not meant to be is just a way to satisfy curiosity, to provide meaning where there isn't any. After many years of learning about psychology, sociology, and human behavior, I've concluded that human beings need answers even if there aren't any, a place to put the blame, a reason for something that has none. For instance, when someone passes away at a young age, a lot of people will say things like God takes the good ones first or it just was/wasn't meant to be (based on the situation). Or if you didn't get the job, lost the big game, got dumped, etc., it's just a way to soften the blows of life with a meaningful nothing. Sometimes we need to accept things as they are regardless of if there's meaning or not.

Now, for those who do believe in a higher power setting our path, yet we have free will, my thoughts don't account for divine guidance. Just because we have free will doesn't mean that your God, the Universe, destiny, etc., doesn't try to guide you through life. It is very possible that divinity has a purpose for you but a purpose that you must come to on your own, like answering a calling, and until you answer that calling, the phone doesn't stop ringing.

The hot take: fate is bullshit. It's just an excuse so you can point the finger when things go bad. To give reason and meaning to situations when there might not be any. But whether I am right or wrong in my assessment makes no difference. You could believe in free will, take control of your life, be aware of your choices and decisions, and if it so happens that we live by destiny's rule, what you've done is what destiny wanted anyway. So, you might as well take responsibility for your own life just in case I'm right.

THE SECRET TO HAPPINESS

Now we get to the fun stuff. Assume I am right about Free Will and you are the one in control of your own life. Simply put, THE ONLY REASON YOU ARE UNHAPPY IS BECAUSE YOU CHOOSE TO BE! Now take a minute to air out your excuses, no time, too much work, family responsibilities, money, friends, life, etc....

All of that, every part of it, is your choice. Maybe you try to please everyone and take too much on, maybe it's poor time management, maybe you just feel stuck and don't know how to get out of it, but whatever the reason, it's still your choice. I get it, it sucks. The truth is you CAN dig yourself out of a hole. So ask yourself, what are you doing about it? What are you doing to change and improve your situation? What are you doing to better yourself? You may have sat and thought about it, only to conclude that you just don't have enough time and or resources. It goes on the shelf with all your other million-dollar ideas. A plan is only good if you're able to implement it. A lot of us (me included) think of these giant elaborate plans that require more than we can give so they aren't obtainable.

Here's the actual secret to happiness... It's accountability! You are where you are based on the choices you've made in life. But that just means you can go wherever you want to go based on the decisions you will make. That includes coming up with an idea, making a plan, breaking the plan down into smaller more manageable steps, and most importantly following through. It doesn't even take all that much effort when you look at the bigger picture. Imagine you want to write a book; what if you wrote a page a day? That seems reasonable, right? By the end of the year, you would have 365 pages. Even if half of it is useless, you'd still have 183 pages of good stuff and 182 pages of ideas or at the very least lessons on what not to write.

When you start being accountable for your choices and actions, something wonderful happens. You get a sense of control. You start to look before you leap. You think twice before doing things. Your time becomes more valuable. And what do most people do with things of value, they protect them, take better care of them, treat them with care and respect. Just like having a fancy sports car you don't want to drive in the snow or rain, or that fancy jewelry you only take out for special occasions. What would happen if you applied that same logic to the most valuable thing in the world, TIME? At the end of the day, only you will value your time the most. Think of when you help a friend. They may be thankful, but why? Because you saved them time by helping, their time to be more specific. When you start to value your time, being accountable becomes easier, prioritizing time becomes easier, setting goals becomes easier, and achieving those goals becomes easier.

Please don't get my words mixed up, when I say it will make things easier, I don't mean things will be easy. They probably won't. First of all, you may need to make sacrifices. Whether it be a night out with friends, your favorite food, or even sleep, they may need to be made to free up some time and/or resources to achieve your goals. Aside from the hurdles that are already in front of you, shit happens. There will be situations that have been thrust upon you. Although you may not always be in control of what happens, you always control what you do next. Being accountable is being aware of the role you played in the cause, effect, and ultimately the solution of any given situation.

The idea here is that despite how hard it will be, the amount of work you'll have to put in, and all the other situations that will try to derail you, staying the course will bring you happiness. That's not to say that you'll feel other emotions on this journey; you most certainly will. But it's okay, you're allowed to. You will fail at times, succeed at others, get mad, be sad, and the list goes on. You may even change your plans along the way. That's ok. You must hold yourself accountable, so if you choose to take a different path, then take it. The most important thing is that it's your choice to do so. It's a lot like playing golf. The conditions are always changing, some days you really aren't that good, other days you're average, and every now and then the wind blows in your favor and you hit the most incredible shot.

The job you have, the friends you keep, and every other situation you find yourself in. It's up to you to decide whether it serves you or hinders you. Stay or go, do or do not, it's always your decision in the end. So do what serves you best!

NOBODY'S PERFECT

But is that a true statement?

Yeah, of course it is, but only with context. Is there one thing in this world that is perfect for everyone? No, there isn't. But are you everyone? No, you're not. So, there are things in this world that are perfect just for you: food, clothing, books, movies, ideas, etc.

There could be the perfect one of any of these things just waiting for you. And if that's a possibility, isn't it possible that there is a perfect person who could provide you with a service: plumber, electrician, lawyer, chef, etc.? And if that's possible, isn't it possible that the perfect life partner could exist, again, just for you? Ergo, you are perfect. But that doesn't mean you shouldn't improve yourself. Learning is a lifelong process, whether it's gaining knowledge, learning a new skill, or becoming healthier, etc. Bettering yourself leads to higher self-esteem. That doesn't take away from the fact that each and every one of us, the way we are, could absolutely be perfect.

The key to all of this is believing in yourself, knowing your strengths and weaknesses, and understanding that there is a big difference between self-esteem and having confidence in oneself. It is perfectly okay to not be confident in one area of life. Can you program a CNC machine, play sports at a professional level, sew your own clothing, paint, cook, ride a bike, swim, etc.? No. Does not being able to do one or many of these things really bother you? Well, you can accept it or learn to do it. Having a good level of self-esteem is realizing that not being confident in a skill doesn't make you any less of a person.

To those who believe perfect doesn't exist, what makes something good enough? Is it 50% of what you want, 60%, 80%? Could this be why no one is ever satisfied? You take what is available until something better comes along. What if you figured out what you want and waited until you got it. Technically, there is no better because you got what is perfect for you. The word perfect doesn't fit anyone or anything globally. It is completely subjective. Your idea of perfection may or may not match anyone else's idea. What's perfect for you is perfect for you. Rather than following trends or taking someone else's advice on what you want, focus on what would serve you best. What meets your needs and requirements. Where in your life you're willing to be open minded and try something new or stick to what you know best. By embracing what serves you best, you empower yourself to lead a more fulfilling life. This means not only considering your immediate desires but also envisioning your long-term goals and aspirations. It's about recognizing that sometimes the path less traveled may lead to unexpected discoveries and growth, while at other times, sticking to what you know best can provide stability and security. By maintaining this balance and staying true to yourself, you cultivate a sense of authenticity and confidence in your decisions. Remember, it's okay to be open-minded and try new things, but it's equally important to honor your instincts and stay grounded in your values. This way, you pave the way for a journey that is uniquely yours, filled with purpose and meaning.

THE ADVICE PARADOX

Everyone has something to say (doesn't mean we actually say it). But when someone shares their problems, most of us immediately put ourselves in their situation and offer our opinion on what should be done, like our version of a solution. Even though we usually have someone's best interest at heart, we really have no idea of the consequences, thoughts, feelings, etc., that will come from our makeshift solution.

The problem with advice is it's based on what we're told. Important details could be missed, forgotten, or even left out on purpose (to shorten the story or just because they're embarrassing to tell). Not to mention how many people take and use someone's advice. Some take it into consideration, others will disregard it completely, and very few will follow it. Overall, the majority of us know or will figure out what is best for ourselves. We have been making decisions since the day we could think for ourselves.

When someone takes your advice, you think you might know better, but based on limited knowledge, it could be completely wrong. You could be partially responsible for someone's failure, and besides feeling bad, it could possibly ruin whatever relationship you had, them putting the blame on you, despite it being their decision in the end. Think about the last time you gave someone advice. What happened? Did they listen to you? What was the outcome of the situation? Ask yourself this, if you were truly in their situation, would you have followed your advice, or is it one of those do as I say, not as I do scenarios?

When you are in a tough situation, how do you make decisions? Are you more emotionally based, or logic based? And when you give advice, are you more emotionally based or logic based? I think it's safe to assume that most of you take your emotions into consideration when deciding for yourself. No one wants to feel bad about the choices we sometimes must make. Also, that's why doing the right thing can be so hard (At least when we are the ones that must do it). But when it comes to advice, logic wins almost every time. Suddenly the hard, right thing to do has become easy and justified. Even if we can understand the feelings they have, the right thing to do is the right thing to do. Maybe we need to take an unbiased approach to this whole advice giving. Instead of just giving someone our best solution (despite not having all the facts and or feelings), we help them think outside the box. Asking questions on how they feel or how they would react if someone came to them with the same problem. Helping them look at the situation from a different perspective. Or even better, saying nothing at all and just listen. A lot of problems aren't even that big, and someone just needs to vent, to be heard, to know they aren't alone. Most people aren't stupid, and there's a good chance they've already thought of whatever you're going to say. What they're hoping for is an easier solution or validation.

We must remember, we aren't them and they aren't us. No matter how well you know someone, to know what their emotional threshold is almost impossible. Most of us don't know our own. At times we can be pushed to the edge only to realize we are able to withstand more. Not everyone can do as you do or think as you think. Not everyone could live with making certain decisions as you could. Next time someone comes to you, be a friend first and just listen.

KILL THEM WITH KINDNESS

It is no secret that having a good attitude leads to being more thoughtful, accepting, and happier. So why are so many people in the world cynical? Always expecting the worst and assuming everyone is out for themselves.

The news and media are mostly to blame. When it really comes down to it, it's about money (Shocker, I know). We as humans are drawn to the terrible, the dangerous, the controversial, etc. News and media companies make money from your attention. In the simplest way of looking at it, more eyes, more dollars. And the best way to keep your attention is to keep you thinking about the dangers of the world, whether it's global, specific to your country, your state or province, or even your city. If you keep coming back for updates, the bank account keeps growing. Hence why you'll see the same stories repeatedly on different news channels, sure to keep you updated, but also to keep you coming back. Once the population is tired of seeing one thing, you'll see a new thing pop up almost like clockwork. All too continuously reassure you that the world is a dangerous place, and you need to keep checking back in for new information on what dangers lurk ahead.

Using a little bit of my own common sense, I find it hard to believe that more "bad" happens in the world than "good". For the most part, we don't live in a chaotic dystopian society (despite what the news may tell us). You don't have to murder, lie, cheat, and steal to survive. We just have this idea that if nothing bad happens, then something bad will. The old saying "No news, is good news" has long been forgotten. We have become brainwashed into thinking that everyone is out to get us and it's only a matter of time. The truth is that's not the case.

Using rounded up figures, the average number of violent crimes in the US in 2021 was about 400 per 100,000 people. That's 0.4% meaning 99.6% of the time nothing happens. Think about that for a minute. You have a less than 1% chance of becoming a violent crime statistic. There is something to be said about living a cautious life but too cautious and you'll have a dark view of the world and more importantly the people in it. Rather than saying hi to a random stranger, we keep to ourselves and don't want to be bothered. If someone smiles at us, we initially think "What does this person want from me", rather than smile back genuinely. We become skeptical if anyone does anything nice for us. I can think of multiple occasions where even holding the door open for someone got me an odd look and reaction rather than a thank you.

The real question is, how do we change this? The simple answer is, be kind! It costs nothing to be polite and grateful. The simplest things like saying "please and thank you" go a very long way. Aside from the fact more people will like you and want to deal with you, you'll get more of whatever it is you want. More people would be inclined to say yes to you knowing that you will appreciate them.

Think of the drive-through employee at your local fast food/coffee shop and the difference between them having a good attitude versus a bad one. How did they make you feel when you got your morning coffee? The cheerful good morning and smile versus someone who barely acknowledges your existence. How does that affect your day? You may think it doesn't do much, but you could be wrong. We all love being acknowledged, and if that put a smile on your face you may go into work happy, maybe you rub off on someone that's having an off morning and improve their day. Then they rub off on someone else, and so on. Maybe we can change the status quo one person at a time by simply being more polite.

It is very hard to ignore something that's right in our faces every day. If I'm kind and you're kind, maybe there are more kind people. Maybe the world isn't as bad as it seems. Even if we stopped right here and this is all you did, your idea of the world would improve greatly. But what if we did a little bit more? Such as killing them with kindness. This is where things get a little more difficult, where you need to dig down deep to see past anger. Understand that most confrontations are misunderstandings and not personal in their nature. So many of us put up walls that when we are challenged, we think someone is trying to invade us. When in reality, they just want to be heard.

Confrontations start because there is a lack of listening, not loud yelling. The tough part is to hear someone out, especially when you don't agree with their sentiment. And if someone doesn't care to hear your side of the story, well then no amount of yelling will get them to. Might as well thank them for their time and opinion and walk away. Focusing on your own inner peace and not allowing others to pollute it. Having a calm demeanor and a reputation for being a good listener will lower the guard of others, leading to more fruitful encounters. The fewer confrontations we have, the less angry we will all be, the less stress we will all carry, the less passing it around to others, and so on.

As I've mentioned before, we are all connected. It all starts with us (as most things do). How kind are you to you? How do you treat yourself? I believe that sets the standard of not only how we treat others but how others treat us. When we allow ourselves to be treated badly, we carry that with us. It affects us mentally, emotionally, physically, and spiritually. Once we learn to be kind to ourselves, it's only natural to be kind to others. When you go to bed tonight, do a quick inventory of your day. How many times were you polite and grateful to someone? How many times did you smile? How many confrontations did you avoid? Regardless of how you think you did, we can all be a little bit better. It's better than being cynical, and it's a lot easier than you think.

THE ART OF LEANING IN

Discovering the Art of Leaning In was a lesson that unfolded later in my life. It's a philosophy that urges one to seize opportunities, embrace the unknown, and expand the boundaries of comfort. At its core, "Leaning In" entails accepting uncertainty, celebrating bravery, and demonstrating the power of courage amidst unpredictability.

The essence of "Leaning In" lies in the willingness to embrace the unknown. Life's twists and turns are inevitable, and despite meticulous planning, derailments are common. Navigating these uncertainties demands adaptability and resilience. Leaning In involves accepting this uncertainty, acknowledging its potential for personal growth, and understanding that fear often holds us back. Yet, by embracing the unknown, we unlock a world of possibilities. While our comfort zone may seem secure, it's often a false sense of security hindering personal development.

Leaning In is essentially about taking risks. Progress seldom occurs without venturing into uncertainty. However, the art lies in assessing risks versus rewards. Courage isn't the absence of fear, but rather the triumph over it. Leaning In necessitates acknowledging fear, understanding its origins, and summoning the strength to move forward despite its presence. It's about discerning which risks are worthwhile and recognizing that the potential rewards outweigh the perceived dangers. Leaning In teaches us to differentiate between reckless impulsivity and calculated risk-taking, urging us to make informed decisions.

While Leaning In doesn't guarantee success, setbacks are inevitable. Resilience becomes crucial in this journey. It's the ability to bounce back from failures, learn from them, and emerge stronger. Resilience acts as a shield, safeguarding us as we navigate uncertainty's turbulent waters. Failures and setbacks aren't reflections of inadequacy but rather opportunities for growth. Leaning In enables us to view challenges not as insurmountable obstacles but as avenues for learning and refinement.

What often impedes progress for many is the fear of failure. However, Leaning In offers a different perspective on failure. Instead of viewing it as an endpoint, it's seen as a checkpoint. Failure, in fact, is life's greatest teacher, imparting invaluable insights rarely gained from success alone. Leaning In challenges the notion that failure should be feared, urging us to embrace it as a natural part of the process, a stepping stone to success. It's about understanding that the road to success is rarely linear but rather a journey marked by detours and setbacks, each offering valuable lessons. Contrary to being a blind leap of faith, Leaning In involves a calculated decision-making process. It requires a delicate balance between intuition and rationality. Intuition serves as a guiding force, nudging us toward decisions aligned with our deeper aspirations, while rationality grounds these decisions in reality. Leaning In entails navigating this balance, trusting our instincts while ensuring our choices are informed by logical reasoning.

Moreover, Leaning In doesn't have to be a solitary endeavor; it can be a collective movement. The art of Leaning In is enriched when individuals come together, sharing experiences, insights, and support. In a community of Leaning In, individuals find strength in shared stories, learning from each other's failures, and celebrating success. This collective energy amplifies the courage needed to embrace uncertainty, making the journey more manageable and rewarding.

Ultimately, the Art of Leaning In serves as a catalyst for personal growth, a journey of self-discovery, self-improvement, and continuous learning. By adopting this philosophy, individuals are invited to dance with uncertainty, confront challenges courageously, and embrace the unknown with open arms. Leaning In isn't recklessness but rather a purposeful pursuit of growth and fulfillment, a celebration of resilience, courage, and the transformative power of embracing life's uncertainties.

AMOR FATI: EMBRACING FATE

Life, with its unpredictability, often presents us with challenges and uncertainties. In such moments, the stoic philosophy of Amor Fati, the love of fate, offers guidance. Amor Fati calls us not only to accept but to embrace our fate, regardless of its nature. It urges us to redefine our relationship with life's struggles, failures, and ordinary occurrences, transforming them into opportunities for growth and self-discovery.

Amor Fati requires a fundamental shift in perspective. Rather than resisting life's challenges, we are encouraged to see them as integral parts of our journey. Every moment, every situation, every obstacle becomes a chapter in our book of life, propelling us forward as we learn and grow.

Applying Amor Fati to our lives grants us the wisdom to recognize that obstacles aren't always what they seem. By embracing this mindset, we gain the resilience to face life's challenges with grace and courage. Not every setback leads to failure, and even those that do offer profound lessons that enrich our lives.

The story of the Chinese Farmer illustrates this concept beautifully.

One day, as the farmer was tending to his crops, his only horse escaped from the stable and ran away. The villagers, upon hearing the news, came to console the farmer for his misfortune. "What bad luck," they lamented, "now you have no horse to help you with your work."

The farmer, however, remained composed. "Good luck? Bad luck? Who knows?" he replied with a serene smile.

Days passed, and to everyone's surprise, the runaway horse returned, leading a herd of wild horses back to the farmer's stable. The villagers, witnessing this unexpected turn of events, rushed to congratulate the farmer. "What incredible luck!" they exclaimed. "Now you have so many horses, you'll be wealthy beyond measure."

Again, the farmer responded with his trademark calmness. "Good luck? Bad luck? Who knows?" he repeated.

In the following weeks, the farmer's son decided to tame one of the wild horses. In the process, he was thrown off the horse and broke his leg. Once more, the villagers gathered to offer their sympathies. "How unfortunate," they murmured, "now your son is injured, and he cannot help you with the farm work."

And once more, the farmer replied, "Good luck? Bad luck? Who knows?"

Shortly after his son's injury, a war broke out in the region. The emperor's soldiers arrived in the village, conscripting all able-bodied young men for the battle. Because of his broken leg, the farmer's son was spared from the draft. The villagers, facing the grim prospect of losing their sons to the war, marveled at the farmer's wisdom. "You are truly blessed," they declared. "Your son's injury saved his life." And as always, the farmer's response echoed through the village, "Good luck? Bad luck? Who knows?"

The story of the Chinese farmer teaches us the profound lesson of embracing the uncertainty of life with composure. What may appear as misfortune in the moment can often lead to unforeseen blessings.

Similarly, in our own lives, setbacks and failures can be opportunities for growth and learning, refining our skills and guiding us toward a brighter future. Amor Fati also teaches us to take responsibility for our lives, empowering us to shape our responses and attitudes toward the challenges we encounter. It encourages a sense of detachment from outcomes, allowing us to focus on the present moment and our responses to it. By embracing uncertainty and detaching from future results, we free ourselves from the paralyzing fear of failure, allowing us to pursue our passions with newfound freedom and purpose.

Moreover, Amor Fati is intertwined with gratitude, a powerful tool that transforms our outlook on life. Gratitude extends beyond acknowledging the positive aspects of life; it encompasses an appreciation for the difficulties that contribute to our growth and resilience. By expressing gratitude for both joyous and challenging experiences, we cultivate strength and resilience, finding solace in the present moment.

In essence, Amor Fati is a transformative mindset that empowers us to live fully, embracing life's uncertainties with courage and gratitude. It invites us to see every moment, every challenge, as an opportunity for growth and self-discovery. By integrating Amor Fati into our daily lives, we embark on a journey toward resilience, gratitude, and a profound love for the unknown.

THE PAST IS A PLACE OF REFERENCE, NOT A RESIDENCE

Have you ever found yourself trapped in your memory's, the weight of regrets, missed opportunities, or unresolved pain? It's a universal struggle, one that often obscures the beauty of the present moment. We must remember the past is a place of reference, not a residence.

Think of your past as a library. It holds valuable lessons, stories, and experiences that have shaped you, but it's not the place to set up camp. This realization is like a gentle nudge, urging you to step out of the shadows and fully embrace the present. Let's face it; carrying the baggage of the past into your present is like trying to sprint with a heavy backpack. Regrets, guilt, and unresolved traumas act as an anchor, holding you back from experiencing the joy and beauty of now. Regrets can be like a song stuck in your head, playing over and over in your mind. But what if you could learn from them? That's the power of acknowledging the past as a reference point. You extract the wisdom without carrying unnecessary burdens. Unresolved guilt and shame are like invisible chains, limiting your capacity for joy. By understanding that the past is a reference, you begin to unlock the gates of self-forgiveness, freeing yourself from the shackles of unwarranted guilt.

For those with past traumas, living in your mind can feel like being stuck in a tornado; we are comfortable in the eye but are too scared to pass through the storm. The truth is healing begins in the present. By acknowledging the past, you create space for understanding, compassion, and the journey toward healing. You will start to realize that it's already happened, and it can't continue to hurt you unless you let it.

But how to use your past as a guide? Using the past as a library of knowledge, where every failure is a lesson.

Here are a few examples.

- Learning from Mistakes: Turning Setbacks into Springboards

    Mistakes are not barriers; they're detours that offer unexpected experiences. By viewing them as a learning experience rather than a reason to nag yourself, you transform your past into a lesson to weigh in on future challenges.

- Celebrating Your Wins

    Successes are like trophies. By reflecting on your achievements, you empower yourself to set ambitious goals with the confidence that you've conquered similar challenges before.

- Embracing Change and Evolution

  Life is a journey, the past are the roads that brought you to this moment. Embrace change as is helps evolve your character.

- Living in the Present

  Looking at the present (the place where you truly reside), living in the now isn't just a philosophy; it's a way of life that can profoundly impact your daily existence, rather than living in the past.

- Mindfulness and Emotional Well-Being

  By being fully aware of your thoughts and feelings, you detach from the chains of the past and find solace in the current moment. This practice has the power to reduce stress, improve emotional regulation, and enhance your overall well-being.

- Nurturing Relationships

  By being fully present with your loved ones, you deepen connections and create shared memories. Living in the past can cast shadows on your interactions. You might be looking for trouble where there isn't any.

- Pursuing Passions and Goals

  Redirect the energy spent dwelling on past failures or anxieties about the future toward actively pursuing what brings you joy and fulfillment. If you want something bad enough, any obstacles in your path will seem like small speedbumps rather than roadblocks.

When you look at the past as a reference, it grants you the power to let go. It's a liberation, a journey toward self-forgiveness, embracing uncertainty, and cultivating gratitude. Forgiveness is not just a gift to others; it's a profound act of self-love. By acknowledging mistakes and forgiving yourself, you create space for self-compassion to flourish. Embracing uncertainty, for it is in the unknown that you discover the beauty of possibility and how your limits once were. Gratitude transforms ordinary moments into extraordinary blessings. By actively appreciating the positive aspects of your life, you shift your focus from what's missing to the abundance you already have. You will never be satisfied if you always focus on what you don't have.

Practical Steps for Living in the Present

Now that we've explored the philosophy of viewing the past as a reference rather than a residence, let's delve into practical steps to help you fully embrace the present moment:

1. Mindfulness Meditation: Start with short mindfulness meditation sessions. Focus on your breath, observe your thoughts without judgment, and gradually extend the duration as you become more comfortable with the practice. Mindfulness meditation cultivates awareness of the present

moment, helping you detach from the chains of the past.

2. Gratitude Journaling: Keep a gratitude journal to actively acknowledge and appreciate the positive aspects of your life. Take a few moments each day to jot down things you are thankful for. Gratitude journaling shifts your focus from what's lacking to the abundance you already possess, fostering a sense of contentment and appreciation.

3. Set Present-Centric Goals: When setting goals, break them down into smaller, manageable tasks that can be tackled in the present. Celebrate each small victory as you progress toward your larger objectives. Setting present-centric goals keeps you focused on the here and now, allowing you to fully engage with the task at hand.

4. Practice Forgiveness: Identify areas in your life where forgiveness is needed, whether directed towards yourself or others. Practice the art of letting go, acknowledging that forgiveness is a gift to your present self. Forgiveness liberates you from the burdens of the past, allowing you to embrace the present with an open heart.

5. Embrace Change: Cultivate a mindset that embraces change as a natural part of life. Recognize that change is the melody of your life's dance, and every step contributes to the beautiful choreography. Embracing change

allows you to adapt fluidly to life's transitions, fostering resilience and growth.

6. Engage in Creative Pursuits: Participate in creative activities that demand your full attention and presence. Whether it's painting, writing, or playing a musical instrument, these endeavors allow you to immerse yourself in the present moment. Creative pursuits unleash your creativity and provide a channel for self-expression.

7. Build Mindful Habits: Turn routine activities into mindful moments. Whether savoring your morning coffee, appreciating the beauty of nature during a walk, or fully immersing yourself in a task at work, these mindful habits enhance your ability to live in the present. Building mindful habits cultivates presence and enhances your overall well-being.

As we conclude this conversation about living in the now, remember this: the past is a library of wisdom, and the present is speeding by right before your eyes. Embrace the past for all that you've been through and the knowledge it has given you, but don't let it trap you. Instead, use that knowledge to guide you through the boundless possibilities of the present. Live with intention, love, and a deep appreciation for the now. As you navigate through life, may you find joy in every step, knowing that happiness is not a destination but a companion on the journey.

THE DUALITY OF MOTIVATION: LIGHT AND DARK SIDE

Motivation, often viewed as a driving force behind our actions, possesses both positive and negative aspects. While it can inspire us to achieve our goals and propel us forward, not all motivations are beneficial. Just as there is light and shadow in the world, motivation also has its bright and dark sides.

Good Motivation: A Beacon of Purpose and Clarity

Good motivation is like a beacon that illuminates our path, providing us with purpose and clarity. Unlike its counterpart, which relies on external validation or fleeting rewards, good motivation emanates from within. It springs from an authentic desire to pursue goals that resonate deeply with our core values and aspirations. Whether it's learning a new skill, making a positive impact on others, or nurturing a personal passion, the intrinsic satisfaction derived from these pursuits transcends material gains. Good motivation is rooted in passion, purpose, and an unwavering commitment to growth and development.

Signs of Bad Motivation: Navigating the Shadows

Conversely, bad motivation lurks in the shadows, vulnerable to doubt, fear, and external pressures. Motivations driven by the need for external validation or fueled by fear often lead us astray. They can cloud our judgment, steer us off course, and ultimately undermine our well-being. When our motivation hinges solely on seeking approval from others or avoiding failure at all costs, it can breed anxiety, dissatisfaction, and a sense of emptiness. Similarly, the pursuit of immediate gratification or goals lacking in genuine meaning or purpose can leave us feeling lost, directionless, and disconnected from our true selves.

Cultivating Good Motivation: Nurturing the Light Within

To cultivate good motivation, we must first embark on a journey of self-discovery and introspection. This involves reflecting on our values, passions, and long-term aspirations. By aligning our goals with our innermost desires and authentic selves, we infuse our pursuits with meaning and significance. Prioritizing personal growth, contribution, and authenticity over external validation allows us to pursue endeavors that resonate deeply with our souls, bringing us a sense of joy, fulfillment, and purpose.

Strategies for Sustainable Success: Illuminating the Path

In our quest to cultivate good motivation, we must equip ourselves with practical strategies and tools to navigate life's twists and turns. Embracing self-compassion, mindfulness, and gratitude empowers us to embrace setbacks as opportunities for growth and learning. By adopting a growth mindset and surrounding ourselves with supportive peers who share our vision and values, we create a nurturing environment conducive to personal and professional development. Setting boundaries to protect our time, energy, and well-being is essential for maintaining balance and avoiding burnout. Visualization techniques can also be powerful tools for harnessing the power of our imagination and channeling it toward achieving our goals.

Motivation is a multifaceted phenomenon that influences every aspect of our lives. By understanding the duality of motivation and cultivating good motivation within ourselves, we can illuminate our path and create a life filled with purpose, passion, and meaning. Motivation serves as both a compass, guiding us toward our goals, and a fuel, sustaining us through life's challenges. Armed with clarity, purpose, and unwavering authenticity, we embark on a journey of self-discovery, growth, and fulfillment.

SECTION 2
SELF FOCUS

SELF-AWARENESS AND SELF-ESTEEM

Self-esteem gives you the ability to do as you wish regardless of who judges you. It is the confidence in your own self-worth. The question is, who is judging you and why are you letting them stop you from doing anything? We have all been there at some point in our life. Whether we are wearing the wrong clothing, playing the wrong sport, liking the wrong music etc. There is only one person whose opinion matters, yourself.

Those with a high level of self-esteem may not understand what that feels like. To them, it comes across as extremely illogical. Why does the opinion of someone stop you from doing anything?

Let's take a logical approach to it. Ask yourself where this person's opinion stems from. Is their opinion based on facts or is it an opinion based on some sort of prejudice? Are they jealous? It could actually be none of the above. The best part is, what all these reasons have in common, none of it matters. As I've already said, the most important opinion that matters is your own. It should supersede all that comes after. You should know if you suck at something and even if you do, does it make you less of a person? NO! If you aren't used to having a high level of self-esteem, it may feel like you're being arrogant when you're used to being passive.

Being assertive may feel like you're being aggressive when you're not used to getting your way. Prioritizing yourself may feel like being selfish. Your comfort zone may not actually be the best benchmark. It is something you'll have to learn to get used to, but being your own person will be liberating. You can finally be yourself. Rather than listening to those who put you down or tell you what to do, you get to enjoy life as you wish to live it. Wear the funky pants, collect stamps, listen to that polka music, whatever puts a smile on your face. As society evolves more and more people are accepted for their differences.

The internet has made the world smaller, meaning it is easier for people to find others who share the same interests. I ask that you do the same if you haven't already. Most groups are excited to find new people who are just like them. You could even make new friends. Despite your self-esteem coming from the inside, it's always nice to be complimented and accepted. Making it easier to be ourselves, be more confident in ourselves, and be prouder of who we are.

The importance of this is life-changing for those who don't already have a high level of self-esteem. So many of us spend time and energy worrying about people accepting us as we are. When we aren't, some try to force change to be something we aren't. Trying to fit someone else's idea of what we should be. When it comes to who we are, those who care don't matter and those who matter don't care. Friends will always offer suggestions just as you will to your friends. Whether those suggestions are taken may define relationships. Do they get mad? Do you get mad when someone doesn't take your suggestions? Being a true friend is about being there for someone, not necessarily forcing them because you think you know better (Obviously there are situations where someone is hurting others or themselves and you want to put a stop to it.). I'm just saying it's okay to be you, it's okay to ask for others to respect you for you (and if they don't it's okay to walk away), and it's okay to enjoy things that might be off the beaten path.

If you happen to be the type of person that loves to give your opinion, especially when it's not asked for, I ask you to have a little self-awareness and be mindful of the impact it may have on someone else. Especially their self-esteem and self-confidence. In a lot of cases, you don't know better and even if you do, it may not be worth the emotional trauma it may cause someone.

MOTIVATION AND PRAISE

Once upon a time, you were a baby (hard to believe, I know). Besides the natural instincts to grab, suck, and sleep, you knew nothing. From that point till now, everything you know and do, you've learned. When you were a baby taking your first steps, what happened? You stood up, someone took notice and called the rest of the family, they all started to cheer you on. When you fell, not a single person said anything bad. They said it's okay, get back up and try again. And you did, one foot in front of the other, you learned how to walk. How about the first time you went potty? They took off your diaper, sat you on the toilet, all for nothing. Time and time again they sat you on that toilet until you pooped. There was a celebration for your ability to poop.

Now let's fast forward to the last time you've had an amazing idea. Maybe it was a little crazy, maybe a lot of work involved, what did your friends and family say? "You're crazy, I mean, it's a good idea, but it probably wouldn't work, there's no way you'd have time for that." And if they said otherwise, you should be very grateful of them. But do you see the pattern, as it seems we are more successful when we have a cheering section. When people believe in us, we believe in ourselves even more and that belief is what gives us the heart and drive to do our best.

We may not succeed, but we will definitely learn. We won't be scared to try again, just like the baby version of us.

Now think back to when a friend or family member had a crazy idea. How did you respond? Did you provide them with some motivation or praise? Now don't get me wrong, a lot of ideas are terrible. But instead of knocking people down, let's give them something to think about and maybe amend, but at the end of it, give them the motivation to keep at it. Hey, you may fail, but you'll never know unless you try. Just like the baby, failure is an option, but without motivation and perseverance, nothing will get done. Side note: don't let someone's lack of expertise deter them from trying.

Professionals think they know it all, but newcomers may think outside the box ideas that may seem impossible and then make them possible. Those are the people that create new technology, invent new things, and find better ways to do almost everything. When we surround ourselves with people that are always negative, it's hard for us to believe in ourselves. When so many people that we respect and trust have no faith in our own abilities, it's hard for us to find motivation. Could they be right? Maybe, but then maybe they're wrong. It might be better to surround yourself with people that also share the same vision as you. Motivation thrives in a positive environment. Surrounding yourself with individuals who see your vision will uplift and encourage you.

Then again, there is always someone you can count on, yourself! After all, it is your idea; it is your life. If you believe strongly enough, then you should pursue.

If you need to find motivation on your own, here are a few ways that could help:

1. At the heart of finding motivation lies purpose. Begin by defining your goals, both short-term and long-term. Understand why it is important to you. The more clarity you have about your goals, the easier it becomes to navigate towards them.

2. Just like walking when you were a baby, you took one step at a time. Goals are achieved the same way. Break down your objectives into smaller, more manageable tasks. This not only makes the process less difficult, but it also provides a sense of accomplishment every time you've completed one of those tasks.

3. Close your eyes and picture your success. Visualization is a tool that aligns your thoughts with your goals. It could even help in creating a mental road map for how to achieve those goals. Envision the joy of reaching every goal. The pride in overcoming the challenges and fulfillment of realizing your dreams.

4. The importance of a routine. Establishing a routine not only creates discipline, but creating a daily schedule that works towards your goals also helps you be consistent. If you're able to be consistent then the process becomes sustainable. Anything that is sustainable has a better chance of being completed.

5. Embrace challenges. Understand that every difficult situation that you come across on your journey is either a path to success or a learning experience and an opportunity for growth. Just like when you were a baby, going from crawling to walking, learning from those challenges will guide your path to success.

Finding motivation must come from within but just like sailing, it's easier on a day with a breeze. Keeping people around you who will support you and help you makes the process much easier. At the end of the day, if you want something bad enough, finding the time, strength, and motivation will seem worth it. Everyone's life is different, even those who share the same vision as you. No one has experienced life as you have. Some people will not understand your reasons but that shouldn't deter you. As much as praise is a nice thing to have, you must always be able to rely on yourself. Your life, your journey, your lessons, your successes, I wish you the best of luck with all of it.

GRATITUDE

"Being thankful for what you have before it's gone"

As the saying goes, "We realize what we have only after it's gone." But why does it have to be that way? Why do we have such a tough time appreciating the here and now, the people who love us, the challenges we overcome? Why do we ignore the good and focus on the bad?

From what I have noticed, greed plays a role in this. And I'm not talking about your typical movie villain stealing candy from kids' greed. It's more of an unspoken, unnoticed, "what I have is not enough" type of greed. One we don't even acknowledge because we feel our lifestyle is in jeopardy. It's troubling if we don't obtain more or at the very least keep what we have. This type of greed could also be associated with fear and anger. We're scared of losing what we have or angry because we didn't get what we want.

But the fact of the matter is, if you were able to afford this book, you are most likely part of the 1% of the world's wealthiest. One-third of the world lives on $2.00 a day. To mildly put that into perspective, you have a lot to be grateful for. In fact, if everyone put their problems into a pile, you would be clawing to have your problems back.

This perspective begs an important question:

How do we live with gratitude each day?

- **Be more polite:** It absolutely takes nothing to be polite and nice to others. Saying please and thank you consistently is at the base of being grateful. You will start to appreciate the sacrifice and kindness of others. If you need to remind yourself why? Would you like to be making everyone else coffee or spending your workday dealing with other people's complaints, probably not, and I'm sure there's a long list of other thankless jobs I could mention. Saying hello or goodbye meaningfully is essentially thanking them for showing up. Smiling is contagious, not to mention a physical act that can change your mood. Smiling makes us feel happy, and being happy makes being grateful easier, and being grateful makes us happier still, like a vicious circle of happiness.

- **Thank yourself:** With life as fast-paced as it is, we tend to take a lot for granted, including ourselves. We all have a lot on our minds, and we even forget to thank ourselves for the sacrifices we've made. So instead of getting lost in our own thoughts, start every day putting the right mindset into place. Every morning, spend some time thinking back to a moment when you were proud of yourself or took the hard high road. Remember why you did it and who you did it for. Realize that by doing so, you made a difference in someone else's life. Reminding yourself of your good-natured deeds may help you see the same in others. Understanding other people will give you the understanding to show them gratitude as well.

- **Keep a gratitude journal:** Take some time and start to write everything you are grateful for and why you're grateful for it. For those tough times in your life, having something to read as opposed to trying to think past your problems is an easy way to take a break from life and be thankful for what you do have. Writing has an effect of making you focus on your thoughts, bringing attention to the subject you are writing about (gratitude in this case). While writing in your journal, consistently describe your thoughts, put yourself back into the memory, feeling the feelings of gratitude and thankfulness, word for word as the encounter unfolds along with the story. Make sure to add what you were feeling and what triggered those feelings. Try to find deeper meaning to why you're feeling and what makes you grateful? Better yet, every time you feel grateful in your daily life, remember to write it down in your journal. The more entries you have, the easier it becomes to be grateful overall.

- **Don't forget the little things:** The habit of gratitude doesn't grow from only feeling grateful from the life-changing instances. Recognizing the little things consciously is a great way to practice the habit of gratitude. A nice day, an extra delicious coffee, even a green light, anything and everything is worthy of being grateful for. Especially if that instance puts a smile on your face. Like everything, practice makes perfect. If it's something you don't already do, it will take some work to adopt it into your daily routine. Bringing focus to the little things in life is a great way to start being thankful.

- **Spend time with those you love**: One of the easiest ways to practice gratitude is to just spend time with friends and family (assuming those are who you love). Having those you love around you will help you appreciate them more. Recognizing that appreciation is gratitude. Do your best to be there for them. Find ways to support them. Instead of itching to tell them your story, listen to theirs. Engage more in their interests showing them you care. Appreciate everything they've done for you. In fact, thank them if you haven't done it already. Let them know how important they are to you by telling them as well as showing them.

As with most things in life, being grateful starts with self-reflection. What contributes to our happiness? What makes life easier? Who makes us feel safe and secure? What, or who puts a smile on our face? Just thinking back and answering these questions alone is a great way to start. Every time you catch yourself smiling, take a second and think about why, acknowledge it, realize who or what to thank. Knowing what made you feel this way makes it easily repeatable. Believe it or not, the benefits of practicing gratitude actually have positive effects on our physical and mental health. Such as, lowering stress, which improves our immune system, eases symptoms of depression and anxiety, which helps us be more optimistic about our present and future life, not to mention improving the relationships we have and will have. If gratitude was on an infomercial, it would almost sound too good to be true: "For only a few minutes a day. You can improve your physical and mental health, your life, your relationships, and your happiness by doing this one thing." Now, doesn't that sound like the deal of a lifetime? And in the end, we don't have to wait for something to disappear before realizing how important it is to us now.

EXPECTATION AND THE THIEF OF JOY

It's only natural for us to get excited when we see or hear that some good is coming our way. A new job, maybe an investment, even the idea of a new partner, but what we sometimes do is jump too far into the future, pre-planning the events in your head as if they will happen exactly as you imagined. Now if it does happen the way you imagined, you are overjoyed, completely filled with happiness. On the other hand, if you were wrong, you could be completely gutted, maybe even depressed. Even if the outcome is still good, it won't feel like it.

Letting your expectations run away with your imagination is much different than overthinking. The difference between the two is that overthinking is like a broad picture of a situation, with many ways it could go, possible outcomes good or bad. Expectations, like the word itself, you're expecting something particular to happen. You're pre-planning and getting yourself emotionally prepared for the outcome. You've already decided how it will unfold. Now, there is something to be said about those who always expect the worst to happen. If the worst happens, then they're prepared. If it doesn't happen then happy days. I'd say that is more like overthinking than expectations. They usually have more than one doomsday scenario and try to prepare for each and every one. Nonetheless, that's not what I'm really talking about here. The point I'm trying to make is not to look so far in advance, but enjoy the moment, the here and now.

Sometimes you have to look at life like a magic trick. Enjoy it for what it is and never mind how it's performed. Time and time again we start to expect more and more until it comes crashing down. Like everything else in this book, it's easier said than done. To learn to focus on what is in front of you instead of what could be. Cherish and enjoy every moment you can, and life might become a tad more pleasant. I know we all get excited when good news is on the horizon. We are all dreamers at heart, right from childhood, pretending we are pilots or astronauts going to the moon.

As we get older, our expectations get a tad more realistic. I would never want to take the joy of dreaming from you, but I do want to remind you the universe owes you nothing. It's 100% up to you to make those dreams real. As great as it feels to let our imagination run up our expectations, it could be robbing us of the joy right in front of our eyes. Expectations can lead us up a cliff that overshadows a pit of despair and depression. You must remind yourself that fantasy isn't worth falling to your doom. Your attention is better utilized getting what you want instead of imagining having what you want, but how to achieve such a thing? Well, like anything in this world, it's going to be different for everyone. I mean, what are you expecting? I'm sure every time in your life you expected something, it was completely different from the last. Something specific for your birthday, the quality of an online purchase, maybe your promotion at work. These examples are not even scratching the surface of the endless possibilities.

But how do you keep your expectations in check?

1. **Look inside yourself:** See where these expectations are coming from. Are we dreaming of this better life? Maybe we watch too many movies and think that's what reality is really like. Could we be comparing ourselves to others? Is it based on things we learned from childhood? The list of sources goes on and on. The important thing is if we know where they're coming from, then maybe we can figure out why we're having them and if they really are realistic. Are we chasing our own dream or the dreams of others?

2. **Ask yourself:** If my expectations were met, would I be happy? If the answer is yes, then it becomes more of a goal, something for you to work towards or find, but at least now you have direction to joy or happiness. If the answer is no, then why expect it in the first place? What gave you the idea to expect this? Since it won't make

you happy, it might be easier to drop and refocus your attention on something more fruitful.

3. **Keep an open mind:** If your expectations aren't met, doesn't necessarily mean it's a bad thing. It could be better than you expected, or different enough that its perceived value will reveal itself at a later time. Hindsight is 20/20. Secondly, we tend to be extremely rigid in our expectations, having an open mind may allow for a bit of flexibility which would allow our expectations to be more easily met.

4. **Forgive yourself:** A lot of the time the expectations we have are placed on ourselves. And a lot of the time, they're beyond our means. Aside from giving ourselves too much work, sometimes it's outside of our control. People, situations, resources can all change in the blink of an eye. If you're honest with yourself and you know that you've done the absolute best you can with what you have, then, you have nothing to be sad or angry about. Forgive yourself, clear your head and live to fight another day.

5. **Share your expectations:** Telling someone you confide in may shed some light if you're being reasonable with your expectations. Think of a time when someone shared their expectations with you. Did you agree they were reasonable? Did you try to reason with them? The value of a trusted friend's perspective could help you

determine if you're being unreasonable. You could also share your expectations with whom you're expecting from. Knowing whether you are able to get what you expect is better than wasting your time. Think of a romantic relationship, is it not better to let the other party know what you're expecting then wasting your time finding out? Being transparent also opens up the lines of communication where your love interest may feel comfortable sharing what they expect of you.

Predicting the unknown is completely impossible. Expectations are you trying to do just that. Because you're so focused on what will happen, you forget to look in front of you to see what is happening. You could be missing out on some amazing things or losing sight of something going terribly awry. Knowing what you want and having goals would be a better alternative to just expecting. That way you have a sense of direction. You can go after what you want and walk away from what you don't, instead of getting whatever comes to you from sitting on your ass wishing or expecting.

WHAT ARE YOU WORTH?

Something is worth only what someone is willing to pay. You're not a something, but someone. Your worth is strictly decided by you. Unfortunately, you can't control how others act or treat people, but what you can do is accept or reject. If someone doesn't treat you the way you find acceptable, you always have the option to walk away. Self-love leads to self-worth. Just as you would give respect, dignity, and trust to someone you love, you should give it all to yourself. Self-worth goes beyond your possessions, your experiences, your successes, and failures. If you stripped all of that away, would you still love you for you? There is nothing wrong with being confident and taking pride in your achievements as long as you don't do these things for love but do them for the love of them.

Regardless of what happens, you are worthy of love, even if you made a mistake or failed. You should always take responsibility for it but remember you made a mistake. That doesn't mean you are a mistake. Apologize if necessary, help correct the issue, and move on. You are not alone. By no means are you the only person experiencing this or who has experienced this. Sharing it with those you love and trust could lead to some insight and at the very least, you'll get it off your chest. Feelings are not meant to be buried, and by letting them out is a form of self-care.

As mentioned, you are not defined by your possessions. The clothes, the car, your bank balance, etc. should bear no weight on your worthiness to others as well as to yourself. Although it being fun to enjoy the finer things in life, we must always recognize that it does not define us. Generally speaking, nothing lasts forever. Money, cars, clothes, even relationships can be gone in an instant. Losing them or not having them to begin with doesn't mean you should see yourself as worthless. You are always worthy if you believe you are.

We all have bad days. We all feel the same feelings. Someone with a high level of self-worth can let them happen, work through them and not let it affect their value to the world. Like everything else, feelings come and go, let them take their course, learn from them, and never feel guilty for having them. If your feelings have you confused, try and reflect on what they are and why you're having them, even if it means taking a break from social norms. If you don't already, you should spend some time alone. I'm not saying become a hermit, but taking time to improve the relationship one has with oneself can be very beneficial. Figuring out your wants, needs, feelings, etc., getting to know yourself better. Having a better relationship with oneself will always lead to a higher self-worth. Think of it in sales terms. If you believe in the product, it helps you sell the product. If you enjoy hanging out with you, then most likely others will too.

Don't sacrifice your well-being, mental or physical health to please others. Others should want to be with you for you and not what you can do for them. If you said no, would they still want a relationship with you? Being able to recognize when you're being used and taken advantage of is key. Is your value based on what you can do or who you are? There is always give and take in every relationship. Understandably some of us give more than we take, maybe it's because we are self-sufficient or don't require a lot. Others take more than they give, and we may even feel someone is being selfish because of it. We may not recognize that quality in ourselves. This is why it's important to know oneself.

Putting yourself first does not make you selfish, although some people may trick you into believing it is. It's about understanding that everybody needs to be able to rely on themselves to put their own needs first. And if someone is relying on you to fulfill their needs, who is really the selfish one? Just as well, if you can't rely on you, how can anyone else? If you can't make yourself happy, how can anyone else? If you can't forgive yourself, how can anyone else? If you can't love yourself, how can anyone else? If you can't see your worth, how can anyone else see your worth?

There is nothing wrong with putting others first. Helping those less fortunate than you is important to your own well-being as well as the well-being of society. The point of this chapter is for you to see your own worth and not let anyone take advantage of you. Don't let people sum you up in a dollar amount or as a service provider. You are a special human being, but you must believe that first!

SHOULD YOU LIE?

NO! But....

Lying is something we all do sometimes, often without even realizing it. But is it ever okay to lie? And what are the consequences of lying?

First of all, let's define what lying is. Lying involves making a false statement or assertion with the intention to deceive or mislead someone. This can include exaggerating, omitting, or twisting the facts. Lying can also be non-verbal, such as faking a smile, nodding in agreement, or pretending to be interested.

There are many reasons why people lie: to avoid conflict, protect themselves or others, gain an advantage, impress someone, escape responsibility, or cope with stress. Sometimes, lying can seem like the easiest or only option in a difficult situation. However, lying can have negative consequences such as damaging trust, hurting relationships, losing credibility, creating guilt, and compromising integrity.

Some argue that lying is justified or necessary in certain situations, like saving someone's life, preventing harm, or upholding a greater good. However, these situations are rare and often involve complex moral dilemmas. In most cases, lying is not the best solution, and there are usually alternative ways to handle situations without compromising the truth.

Consider this scenario: Dan and Nora are dating casually, but Nora wants to be exclusive. She hints at this to Dan, but he doesn't seem to get it. So, she keeps her options open and goes on a date with John. While on her date, she ignores Dan's messages. Later, she replies and says goodnight. The next day, Dan asks what she did last night. Nora says she was out with a friend. Dan doesn't ask any more questions and lets it go.

Did Nora lie? Technically, no. She didn't make a false statement, but she withheld information relevant to Dan. She implied her friend was not a romantic interest, which was misleading. This is called a lie of omission and can be just as harmful as a lie of commission. By not being honest with Dan, Nora risks their relationship and her own happiness. She disrespects Dan's right to know the truth and make his own decisions. If Dan finds out the truth, he may feel betrayed, hurt, and angry. He may also question everything else she has said or done. Nora may feel guilty, conflicted, and insecure about her choices, losing Dan's trust, respect, and possibly his love.

What could Nora have done differently? She could have been clearer and more direct with Dan about her expectations and feelings, asked how he felt about their relationship, and expressed her desire for exclusivity. Rather than dating someone else, she could have been honest with herself about what she truly wanted and needed from a relationship.

White lies are small, harmless lies we tell to spare someone's feelings, avoid awkwardness, or be polite. For example, we may compliment someone's cooking even if we don't like it, say we're busy when we're not, or claim to like someone's gift when we don't. We may think these lies are harmless and even beneficial, but are they really?

White lies can have unintended consequences. They can reinforce undesirable behavior, erode trust and authenticity, and create more lies. For instance, if we tell someone their cooking is great, they may continue making the same dish or think they don't need to improve their skills. They may feel disappointed or embarrassed if they find out we didn't like it, losing confidence in their abilities and in themselves. If we lie about small things, people may wonder what else we're lying about, doubting our sincerity and honesty, and feeling hurt or offended if they discover our lies. This can lead to a loss of respect and the perception that we don't care enough to tell the truth. Additionally, lying once can lead to more lies to cover up the previous one, creating stress, anxiety, cognitive dissonance, guilt, and shame.

The best way to avoid white lies is to be honest but also kind and respectful. We can use constructive feedback, empathy, and tact to deliver the truth in a helpful, not hurtful, way. Offering suggestions, alternatives, or solutions can also be beneficial. Trusting that the other person can handle the truth and appreciate our honesty, and respecting ourselves and our values by being true to ourselves and others, are key. For example, if someone asks how we like their cooking and we don't like it, we can say: "I appreciate your effort and generosity, but this dish is not really to my taste. Maybe you could try a different recipe or spice next time. I'm sure you can make something delicious." This way, we're honest but also polite and supportive, giving them a chance to improve and learn from their mistakes.

Understanding why people lie can help us empathize and forgive them. Here are some common reasons: to avoid punishment, gain monetary value, protect oneself or others from physical harm, gain popularity, or gain power or control over others. For example, people may lie to avoid punishment when they know they've done something wrong, whether it be an honest mistake or something intentional. This can help us understand their motives and forgive them. Some lie to gain monetary value, like scam call centers, while others, like a kid lying on a resume to get a job, are just looking for a chance. While still wrong, the latter is easier to forgive. Lying to protect oneself or others from physical harm is perhaps the most understandable and acceptable reason to lie. However, lying to gain popularity or control over others, such as creating fictitious stories or manipulating information, is always wrong and harmful.

The worst type of lying is lying to oneself, which hinders personal growth and prevents us from seeking help or expanding our knowledge. We lie about being hurt physically or mentally, stopping us from getting help and making the damage worse. We lie about topics, thinking we know everything, which prevents learning more or considering different opinions. Lying to ourselves prevents accountability, which is essential for happiness. Being honest with ourselves is the first step to accepting ourselves.

Lying is a common and complex behavior with various motives and consequences. While some lies may seem harmless or even beneficial, they can cause harm and distrust. The best way to avoid lying is to be honest but also kind and respectful. Understanding and empathizing with why people lie can help us forgive them. Being honest with ourselves and accepting ourselves for who we are allows us to live with peace, joy, and freedom.

FEAR AND THE PURSUIT OF ACCEPTANCE

In the journey toward self-improvement and personal growth, there is a constant tug-of-war between our fear of rejection and our desire to be accepted. Fear, in its countless forms, often masquerades as a barrier to our authentic expression. It whispers doubts into our minds, convincing us that if we reveal our true selves, we'll face rejection and ridicule. This fear stems from a primal instinct for survival—our ancestors relied on group acceptance for protection and nutrition. However, in today's world, this fear often manifests as anxiety, insecurity, and a relentless pursuit of external validation.

To begin to overcome your fears, you must first identify them. Take time to pinpoint the specific fears that are holding you back from being authentic. Are you afraid of judgment, rejection, or failure? Try to understand the root cause. For example, if you fear rejection, reflect on past experiences that may have contributed to this fear and challenge any irrational beliefs associated with it. Question the validity of your fears: Are they based on actual evidence or inaccurate perceptions? Challenge negative beliefs with rational thinking and positive affirmations. For instance, if you fear failure, remind yourself of past successes and the lessons learned from perceived failures. Replace self-defeating thoughts with empowering beliefs that affirm your worthiness and resilience.

Simultaneously, the desire to be accepted runs deep within our psyche. From childhood, we seek approval from parents, peers, and society. This desire drives us to conform to societal norms, even at the expense of our authenticity. We fear being singled out and not accepted for being different. Therefore, we wear masks, hiding our true selves to fit in.

To live authentically, clarify your core values and beliefs. What truly matters to you? By aligning your actions with your values, you can attract like-minded individuals into your life. For example, if integrity is a core value, stick to your principles even if it means standing apart from the crowd. Establish healthy boundaries to protect your authenticity. Learn to say no to situations or relationships that compromise your values. Practice assertiveness and communicate your boundaries with clarity and respect. For instance, if a friend consistently disrespects your boundaries, calmly but firmly state your needs and expectations in the relationship. If they aren't met, perhaps that relationship isn't worth your time and energy. Don't be afraid to walk away from situations that compromise your sense of self.

Embracing authenticity requires navigating the delicate balance between fear and the desire for acceptance. It involves peeling back the layers of social conditioning and reclaiming the essence of who we truly are. True authenticity doesn't guarantee acceptance; it invites vulnerability, opening us up to the possibility of rejection. However, it also paves the way for genuine connections rooted in mutual understanding and respect.

Take time to practice self-expression. Engage in activities that allow you to express your true self, whether through art, writing, or music. Embrace your unique talents and interests without fear of judgment. Experiment with different forms of self-expression and find outlets that resonate with your authentic voice. For example, if you enjoy writing, start a journal or blog where you can freely express your thoughts and emotions. Surround yourself with people who encourage and accept you as you are. Join groups with like-minded individuals who share your passions, fostering authentic friendships based on mutual respect and understanding.

Being authentic begins with self-acceptance. Acknowledge your strengths and weaknesses, embracing both the light and shadow aspects of your being. Practice self-compassion, recognizing that differences are an inherent part of being human. Release the need for external validation and find validation within yourself. Treat yourself with kindness and compassion, especially during times of self-doubt. Practice positive self-talk and affirmations—the more you say it, the more you'll believe it. Treat yourself as you would a close friend, offering empathy and understanding in moments of vulnerability.

For example, if you make a mistake, acknowledge it without harsh self-judgment and focus on learning from it instead. Celebrate your achievements, no matter how small. Focus on your progress and growth rather than comparing yourself to others. Keep a gratitude journal where you write down your accomplishments and what you're most thankful for. Celebrate your unique talents and recognize the value you bring to the world.

Authenticity requires vulnerability. If you want to be seen and heard, flaws and all, you must embrace vulnerability. Share your truth with courage and conviction. True intimacy arises from genuine self-disclosure and complete transparency. Understand that not everyone will like you, and that's okay. Surround yourself with individuals who appreciate you for who you are. Engage in open and honest communication with others, expressing your thoughts, feelings, and needs. Be willing to listen with empathy and compassion, creating a safe space for mutual vulnerability. Practice active listening, focusing on understanding the other person's perspective without judgment or interruption. Wait your turn to share your own experiences and emotions. Step outside of your comfort zone and take calculated risks that align with your desires and goals. Challenge yourself to try new things and pursue opportunities that inspire and excite you, even if they involve some level of risk or discomfort. Trust in your abilities and intuition, knowing that every experience, whether positive or negative, contributes to your personal growth and development.

In the pursuit of self-improvement and personal growth, authenticity is the foundation upon which genuine fulfillment is built. Release the grip of fear and the desire for acceptance. Embrace your true self with courage and conviction, knowing that authenticity is the key to unlocking a life rich in meaning and connection. Be unapologetically yourself, for in embracing your authenticity, you'll find true acceptance not from others, but from yourself.

SECTION 3
HABITS

DONE IS BETTER THAN PERFECT

I want to share a piece of wisdom that has profoundly impacted my life: "Done is better than perfect." While perfection sounds ideal in theory, in practice, chasing perfection often yields diminishing returns.

How many times have you found yourself endlessly refining a project, trying to achieve perfection? How many projects have you abandoned because the pursuit of perfection burned you out? Perfectionism is generally unattainable not because you can't achieve what you want, but because what you want constantly evolves. As you work, new ideas flood your mind, tempting you to add, change, or modify what you've already done.

"Done is better than perfect" reminds us that sometimes good enough truly is good enough. It gives us permission to let go of the need for perfection and move on to the next project. Done means progress, momentum, and forward movement toward your goals. From this perspective, done actually means perfect.

Perfectionism can be a significant stumbling block on the path to personal growth and success. Constantly striving for perfection can trap you in a cycle of endless refinement, making the prospect of starting new projects daunting. The more you chase perfection, the more it becomes an obsession—a mirage you can never reach. In the process, you miss out on the joy of the journey and the satisfaction of a job well done, even if it's not perfect.

Embracing the idea of getting things done frees you from the shackles of unattainable standards. It allows you to be human, to make mistakes, and to learn and grow from those mistakes. Letting go of the need to be perfect opens up a world of possibilities. You become more resilient, adaptable, and creative, no longer afraid to take risks because you understand that failure is not the end of the world—it's just a stepping stone to success.

This doesn't mean you should abandon all standards and settle for the bare minimum. There's a difference between striving for excellence and chasing an unattainable ideal. Set realistic goals for yourself, break them down into manageable tasks, and celebrate your achievements, no matter how small. It's okay to make mistakes—more than okay, it's necessary.

When you focus on progress, you become more productive and less stressed. You're no longer held back by the fear of making mistakes or falling short of your expectations. Instead, you're moving forward, taking one step at a time toward your goals. The more you focus on progress, the closer you get to a realistic, achievable form of perfection that comes from continuous improvement and a willingness to learn and grow.

How much self-compassion do you have? Do you often beat yourself up over mistakes or shortcomings? Do you hold yourself to a higher standard than you would a friend? It's time to change that. Be kind to yourself. Treat yourself with the same compassion and understanding that you would offer a friend. When you make a mistake, acknowledge it, learn from it, and move on. Remember, you are worthy of love and acceptance exactly as you are.

Self-compassion is not about excusing bad behavior or avoiding responsibility. It's about recognizing your humanity and treating yourself with kindness and understanding. The next time you dwell on a mistake or berate yourself for not being perfect, take a deep breath and remember you are doing the best you can with the knowledge and resources you have in this moment and that's enough.

Perfection is a moving target, influenced by new knowledge, different perspectives, or standards that may be entirely unattainable. In reality, done isn't just better than perfect, done is perfect. Finish your projects, then set new goals and parameters to make them better. This iterative process is how most programs, apps, and products are developed. It's no coincidence that new versions of phones or cars come out each year they are finished, then improved. Set realistic goals, complete them, and move on to the next.

BE CAREFUL OF WHAT YOU WANT BECAUSE YOU MIGHT JUST GET IT

I want to start off by telling you a story about a friend who asked me for dating advice.

In my late 20s, this girlfriend of mine (we'll call her Jane) would always complain to me about the state of men. None of them are serious, or not established enough, or just wanted sex, etc. Until one day Jane met John. John was an above average looking guy, somewhat tall, fit-ish, a soft speaker, stable career, etc. On paper, John would be more than perfect to a ton of women, but he had his eye on Jane. It wasn't long before the two of them became a couple. And maybe a year and a half after that, he proposed. Of course, she said yes, but not coming to me beforehand.

She told me she suspected he was going to propose. I gave her my early congratulations. She was so fixated on finding a good guy she could have a family with, a good provider, potential father, etc. I was so happy for her, she found exactly what she was looking for. All those bad dates finally paid off. As she tells me about her suspicions of a marriage proposal, she mentions to me the feeling of something missing. She described it as that feeling when you go on vacation and know you forgot something but have no idea what. She said it started when they were getting pretty serious, and this feeling has only gotten worse.

This had me very intrigued. "Any idea what it could be?" I asked.

She was pretty much clueless. She told me he's like the perfect guy and she was pretty sure she loved him. I said, "Pretty sure? You do know marriage is for life in a matter of speaking."

She replied, "Sure enough, I guess, he just has everything I want."

To which I said, "Everything except the one thing you don't even know you're missing. If you're unsure maybe you should figure it out before your wedding day."

She assured me she'd try. I don't think she did, because not even a few weeks later, he did propose, and not too long after they got married. For years we never talked about that night and that feeling she had. Like the conversation never even happened. Until one night at 2:00 AM about 10 years after that conversation my phone rang. Jane sounded very sad, almost crying. I right away asked what's wrong as she's never called me this late. She proceeded to tell me that feeling never went away and instead got much worse. She said when they had kids the feeling subsided but as her kids got older, that feeling crept back up, getting stronger and stronger. She felt she might have made a mistake marrying this guy. What makes it worse is that he is an incredible husband and father, so why did she feel this way?

Obviously, I have no idea, but from what it sounds like, her husband was a one, not the one. I assumed that extra something that was missing was the spark, but that spark was never there. She was so fixated on finding someone that could provide her with a family and stable life she forgot to include the importance of the spark. Unfortunately, she had made her bed and now must sleep in it.

In the journey of life, sometimes we get exactly what we ask for. But what if what we thought we wanted isn't truly what fulfills us? How do we navigate the maze of desires to uncover our genuine aspirations?

In our quest for fulfillment, we often chase illusions of what we believe will make us happy. Take the story of a woman who sought a husband and a great father, rather than the love of her life. This classic example reminds us that sometimes, what we think we want may not align with our deepest desires.

The first step towards uncovering our true desires is to be brutally honest with ourselves. We must confront our shortcomings, acknowledge our strengths, and embrace our authentic selves. Only then can we embark on a journey of self-discovery with clarity and purpose.

Too often, we let fear hold us back from pursuing our true desires. Whether it's concerns about cost, societal judgment, or readiness, these fears inhibit our ability to live authentically. But what if we dared to want without reservation? What if we let go of the fear and embraced our desires wholeheartedly?

Reflection is a potent tool on the journey to self-discovery. By setting aside time each week to ponder our experiences and emotions, we gain valuable insights into our evolving desires. Keeping a journal allows us to track our growth over time, providing a roadmap for our journey forward.

In a world filled with endless desires, prioritization is key. We must learn to discern what truly matters to us and focus our energy accordingly. While everything may be achievable, we must recognize that it's rarely possible to pursue all our desires simultaneously.

When faced with uncertainty, it's essential to approach the problem from different angles. By identifying what we don't want and why, we can uncover clues that lead us closer to our true desires. This process of exploration and self-discovery opens doors to new possibilities and paves the way for personal growth.

In the journey of life, understanding your true desires is a voyage that demands courage, honesty, and introspection. It's about peeling back the layers of superficial wants to uncover the core of what will bring you genuine fulfillment. Remember, the pursuit of self-knowledge is not a destination but a continuous journey. Along this path, you'll encounter trials and triumphs, each offering valuable lessons and insights. By embracing this odyssey with an open heart and a reflective mind, you'll navigate towards a future brimming with purpose and joy. So, take a step forward, not in haste, but with deliberate strides, knowing that each step is a step closer to the life you aspire to lead.

WHAT YOU WANT VS WHAT YOU WANT TO WANT

Understanding the nuanced difference between what you want and what you truly desire is pivotal in shaping a life of purpose and fulfillment. At first glance, the distinction may seem subtle, but upon deeper reflection, it reveals profound implications for personal growth and contentment.

What you want often stems from immediate impulses a desire for indulgence, gratification, or conformity to societal norms. It manifests as the impulse to splurge on weekend outings with friends, the allure of the latest technological gadgets, or the craving for trendy fashion items. These desires are often driven by external influences such as advertisements, peer pressure, or societal expectations.

On the other hand, what you want to want represents a deeper, more introspective level of desire, an alignment with your core values, long-term aspirations, and authentic self. It transcends fleeting impulses and requires a deliberate examination of your innermost desires and priorities. It encompasses aspirations for personal growth, health and well-being, financial stability, and meaningful relationships.

To bridge the gap between these two realms requires a conscious commitment to align your actions with your true desires. It begins with introspection—taking the time to reflect on your desires, motivations, and values. Start by making a list of your wants and examining the underlying reasons behind them. Ask yourself why you desire certain things and whether they truly align with your long-term goals and values.

For example, you may find yourself craving the latest smartphone, but upon deeper reflection, you realize that what you truly desire is financial stability and freedom from materialistic pursuits. This realization prompts a shift in perspective, leading you to prioritize saving and investing in experiences that enrich your life rather than accumulating possessions.

Once you've identified your true desires, the next step is to take deliberate action towards realizing them. This requires discipline, commitment, and a willingness to step outside your comfort zone. For instance, if you aspire to lead a healthier lifestyle, you might commit to regular exercise, mindful eating, and prioritizing self-care over indulgent habits. Surrounding yourself with supportive individuals who share similar values and goals can significantly enhance your journey towards aligning your actions with your true desires. Seek out mentors, join communities, or enlist the support of friends and family members who can provide encouragement, accountability, and guidance along the way.

Moreover, imagining someone you deeply respect observing your actions can serve as a powerful motivator to stay aligned with your true desires. Consider how your choices and behaviors would be perceived by this individual and strive to live up to their expectations. Hold yourself accountable for your actions and choices and be willing to course-correct when necessary.

Inevitably, the journey towards aligning your wants with your true desires will be filled with challenges, setbacks, and moments of self-doubt. Embrace these obstacles as opportunities for growth and learning, and remain steadfast in your commitment to living authentically.

By consciously navigating the divide between what you want and what you truly desire, you embark on a transformative journey towards a life of purpose, fulfillment, and authenticity. Embrace your true desires, take deliberate action, and cultivate a life that reflects your deepest values and aspirations. In doing so, you not only enrich your own life but also inspire others to pursue their true desires and live authentically.

ROME WASN'T BUILT IN A DAY

Rome wasn't built in a day, and it wasn't built by one person. From the day we are born, there are people taking care of us (Whether they do a good job or not is another story). As we transition from childhood to adolescence and then to adulthood, there are individuals who accompany us along the way. No matter how much we may believe we've achieved independently, we've always received assistance. What I'm emphasizing is that everything requires time and support from others, whether directly or indirectly. Every lesson we've learned has someone to thank. Consider this book, for example. I must express gratitude to all those who have prompted me to contemplate life, love, and happiness, including the authors of the books I've read on navigating life and emotions. I also appreciate those who have challenged me, as their actions have pushed me to aspire for better. Each influence is akin to a brick in the construction of the Roman Empire. Reflecting back to the day of my birth, as much as I acknowledge it all, I realize I should be more proactive in expressing thanks to those who have contributed to my journey. I encourage you to take a few minutes each day to contemplate those who have supported you and consider how you can express gratitude and appreciation towards them. Throughout this book, I've reiterated the importance of living with gratitude for inner peace. By cultivating inner peace, you can better focus on what truly matters.

Let's dissect this into two parts: time and assistance.

Patience is indeed a virtue, and it's not to be underestimated. We often overlook the value of patience in today's fast-paced world, where we're accustomed to the instant gratification offered by the Internet and services like Next Day Shipping. This mindset has permeated into people's daily lives. For instance, someone secures a new job and within weeks, they're already seeking a raise or an extended vacation. Or in relationships, individuals experience intense feelings and immediately envision marriage on the horizon. I often feel compelled to shake people by the shoulders and implore them to just relax. We're forgetting the joy of anticipation, like eagerly awaiting Christmas morning to unwrap our presents or simply enjoying the company of a special someone without fixating on what comes next. We've become obsessed with the idea of instant recognition for our efforts, whether it's a promotion or acknowledgment from others. Yes, waiting can be frustrating at times. However, the lesson it teaches us is invaluable. It forces us to reflect on whether we truly desire something or if we are looking to give in to impulse. If we genuinely want or need something, it's usually worth the effort and the wait. Consider instances in your own life where your impatience's led to you being disappointed. Life continued, and you found peace nonetheless, realizing perhaps you didn't want it as much as you thought. Some of you may still find yourselves patiently waiting for something, questioning whether to continue to wait or cut your losses and move on. I wish I could help you with that, but that decision lies solely with you. Take a moment to step back, evaluate the situation, and ask yourself if it's truly worth it. Don't give up to easily, but also don't linger indefinitely.

Depending on your personality, requesting or receiving help can prove exceedingly challenging. If you're someone who can comfortably seek and accept help, congratulations (This part may not be for you). However, for those grappling with substantial ego issues, it's time to pause and reconsider. Without assistance, be it direct or indirect, you wouldn't be reading this book today. As previously mentioned, someone had to nurture you, educate you, and guide you along the way. And let's not forget, learning is a lifelong journey that necessitates someone to impart knowledge, whether through written materials, instructional videos, or experiential learning. Consider the age-old trope of a man refusing to ask for directions and instead aimlessly drive around. While the invention of GPS may have altered the literal interpretation, the underlying message remains relevant. Perhaps you're not lost on the road, but rather lost in life. While I may be taking a somewhat extreme stance, I firmly believe this is a critical issue to address. Does seeking help diminish your worth as a person? Does it signify failure? On the contrary, true failure lies in giving up. Seeking help signifies acknowledgment and readiness to receive assistance. Perhaps you're among those who adamantly believe you don't require assistance. You've navigated life for years, possibly decades, with your own methods. I urge you to challenge this belief. Think back and ask yourself if there were times where you thought you were right and weren't, or times you just walked away and didn't know exactly why.

If you've found yourself repeatedly asking "why me?" or struggling with addictive behaviors or anger management issues, it's time to seek professional help. Just as you would see a doctor for pain or taking your car in for making a funny sound. Our brains and emotions can also be worked on. And with everything else, the more you maintain it, the longer it lasts without problem. The reasons to consider therapy are myriad, extending far beyond the scope of this book. Perhaps it's time for all of us to check in with a therapist to assess our ability to cope with life's challenges.

Patience is an incredibly valuable ally. It assists us in discerning if something is truly suitable for us, in evaluating our genuine desires, and even in avoiding pitfalls like consuming undercooked chicken. However, being patient doesn't imply that we should always wait. Rather, it advocates for a more contemplative approach to life, urging us to assess if something merits our patience and commitment. When it comes to seeking help, the adage "two heads are better than one" holds true. Collaboration often yields superior outcomes, just as four hands are better than two. Navigating life with gratitude for all those who directly and indirectly help us may aid us in our thinking. If we recognize the help we've received and the lessons we've learned, it makes it easier to grow as a person and even potentially ask for help in the future.

ONLY DEAD FISH GO WITH THE FLOW

"Only dead fish go with the flow" encapsulates a profound truth about human nature: the danger of passiveness and drifting aimlessly through life without purpose or direction. While the phrase sounds catchy, its implications run deep, touching on themes of autonomy, accountability, and the pursuit of personal fulfillment.

At its core, this phrase warns against the pitfalls of conformity—surrendering one's will to the whims of the crowd. There's an allure to blending seamlessly into society without causing disruptions. It's often easier to agree with others than to swim against the current and risk being labeled a troublemaker. But this surrender of autonomy can lead to losing ourselves, becoming mere bystanders in our own lives. We allow external forces to dictate our choices and shape our destinies, leading to a subtle form of self-betrayal and a gradual erosion of our individuality.

This detachment from our desires can have profound consequences. While it may feel comforting to defer to others' judgment, this behavior can lead to a profound sense of disconnection from ourselves, leaving us feeling adrift and unfulfilled. Moreover, by handing over responsibility for our choices, we miss out on opportunities for growth and self-improvement. It's easy to blame external factors when things don't go our way, rather than acknowledging our role in shaping our circumstances. True personal development requires confronting our shortcomings, taking ownership of our actions, and learning from our mistakes. Accountability is key: when we go with the flow, we forfeit responsibility for our decisions, becoming passive observers in our own lives.

This doesn't mean going with the flow is always wrong. There are times when deferring to the collective wisdom or trusting others' judgment is wise. But it's crucial to do so mindfully, with a clear understanding of our values and priorities. It's about balancing flexibility and assertiveness, adapting to changing circumstances while staying true to ourselves. There's an art to going with the flow without losing sight of our goals. It requires self-awareness and emotional intelligence, knowing when to assert ourselves and when to yield. Life is dynamic and ever-changing, and our path may not always be clear or straightforward. Going with the flow can be seen as an active surrender, a willingness to embrace uncertainty and trust our intuition. It's a leap of faith that can lead to greater clarity and self-discovery.

The most dangerous aspect of going with the flow is the risk of complacency, settling for a life of mediocrity and missed opportunities. Passively drifting through life robs us of the chance to pursue our passions and chase our dreams. We become like dead fish, floating aimlessly in the current, content to let life pass us by. This is why it's essential to cultivate a sense of agency and purpose, actively seeking growth and self-improvement. Taking charge of our destiny means charting a course that reflects our deepest values and aspirations, embracing life's inherent uncertainty, and turning it into a source of strength rather than fear.

The next time you find yourself tempted to go with the flow, pause and reflect on what it truly means. Ask yourself if you're surrendering out of fear or convenience, or if you're making a conscious choice to embrace the unknown and trust the journey ahead. Only by taking ownership of our choices and embracing life's fullness can we avoid becoming like dead fish, doomed to drift endlessly in the currents of fate.

HOW MUCH ARE YOU WILLING TO TAKE?

Life often presents us with challenges that push us to our limits. Whether it's in our jobs or relationships, we sometimes wonder how much we can take before we decide to make a change. This is what we call the Region-Beta Paradox; it's the idea that we can bounce back from tough situations better than we can from ones we just put up with. Imagine you're deciding how to get somewhere. If it's close, you might walk. But if it's far, you'd probably drive because it's faster. It's safe to say we would go farther faster based on this presumption. The same idea applies to life challenges—the tougher they are, the more determined we become to overcome them.

Let's look at an example: you might have a job where most days are okay, but some are really tough. You stick with it because that's what you're supposed to do, right? Work isn't supposed to be fun. But then there's John. John has a terrible job, gets harassed constantly, and comes to find out that similar positions at other companies pay significantly more. Instead of just putting up with it, he decides to find a better job and he does.

John's story shows us that reaching our breaking point can sometimes be the push we need to change for the better. But why wait until things get unbearable? Take a step back and think about your situation. Are you truly happy? Could there be a better path for you?

This isn't just about work it's about every part of our lives, including relationships. Sometimes we settle for things that aren't great but aren't terrible either. But if we take a closer look, we might realize that we deserve better. So ask yourself: Could I be happier? Could my relationships be more fulfilling? Could I improve my life in any way? The answers might surprise you, but they're important to consider if you want to grow. To make positive changes, we need to be aware of our situation and take responsibility for our happiness. If we're unhappy and do nothing about it, we're only holding ourselves back.

Embrace the Region-Beta Paradox as a reminder that we're capable of overcoming tough situations and finding happiness on the other side. Don't be afraid to step out of your comfort zone; it's where real growth happens. Take control of your life and chase after the future you deserve. The journey starts with a single step towards a brighter tomorrow. But let's delve deeper into the intricacies of the Region-Beta Paradox. Think of it as a mental resilience muscle the more we exercise it, the stronger it becomes. Each challenge we face, whether big or small, is an opportunity to strengthen this muscle. And just like any other muscle in our body, it requires consistent effort and practice to reach its full potential.

Consider the concept of comfort zones. We all have them those familiar, cozy spaces where we feel safe and secure. But as comforting as they may be, they also serve as barriers to growth and self-discovery. The Region-Beta Paradox urges us to venture beyond these confines, to embrace discomfort as a catalyst for transformation.

Think back to a time when you were faced with a daunting challenge a moment when you felt like giving up was the only option. What did you do? Did you succumb to the weight of despair, or did you summon the courage to persevere? Chances are, you emerged from that experience stronger and more resilient than before. Now imagine applying that same mindset to every aspect of your life. Instead of settling for mediocrity, you strive for excellence. Instead of shying away from adversity, you embrace it as an opportunity for growth. This shift in perspective can be truly liberating, empowering you to break free from the shackles of self-doubt and complacency.

But let's not forget the importance of self-awareness and accountability in this journey of self-discovery. It's not enough to simply recognize the need for change we must also take decisive action to bring about that change. Whether it's setting goals, seeking support from loved ones, or seeking professional guidance, every step we take brings us closer to realizing our full potential.

The Region-Beta Paradox serves as a powerful reminder of our innate capacity for resilience and growth. By embracing discomfort and pushing beyond our perceived limits, we unlock new realms of possibility and potential. So the next time you find yourself faced with a daunting challenge, remember this: within every setback lies the seed of opportunity. It's up to you to nurture that seed and watch it bloom into something truly extraordinary.

GAMBLING YOUR FUTURE HAPPINESS: THE SUNK COST FALLACY

Let's say you take a new job. It doesn't pay as much as your old job, but you are promised more in a matter of months as well as an opportunity to grow with the company. Six months go by, and nothing happens. No raise, no promotion. A year goes by, and still no raise, no promotion. So you decide to ask management some questions. They still promise you the world. You put your head down and keep working hard.

You start dating someone new. You're crazy about them, but they partake in recreational drugs from time to time. You didn't really have a problem with that before, but now it bothers you. They promise they'll stop, but instead it gets worse. You bring it to their attention, and they promise it will stop again, but nothing changes.

The question is, at what point do you cut your losses?

If you're not familiar with the sunk cost fallacy, it is "the phenomenon whereby a person is reluctant to abandon a strategy or course of action because they have invested heavily in it, even when it is clear that abandonment would be more beneficial." It tends to be easier to notice when it's about financial investment, but when we're talking about people or relationships, it's way harder to notice.

Over the course of my life, I've become the guy people come to for advice, especially dating advice. Time and time again, friends call and ask what they should do next. Despite the first date not going well, or the second, or even the third, they keep seeing something that wasn't there. They say they spend so much time going on dates and talking to these specific people. They feel that something would change. But this isn't someone they've been dating for years. This is brand new, and all interactions were at best meh. I get it. They were sold a bill of goods, and they're waiting for those goods to bear fruit. In one of these situations, a girlfriend of mine spent a year and a half waiting, telling me the whole time that she knew he wasn't the one. But yet she stuck it out for that long. It took a year and a half to figure out that he wasn't who she thought he was.

At what point do you walk away from something and cut your losses? I wish I could tell you there's an easy way to figure it out, but there isn't. This is one of those times you'll have to dig really deep and look at everything as a whole. Is what you're doing helping you reach the goal you're trying to achieve? Is the situation becoming more stressful than it's worth? Are you starting to feel it's a big waste of time? Is it affecting other parts of your life?

Deciding to walk away has its own set of challenges. You will be emotional, for better or worse. Even if you think you're solid as a rock, there's no telling what you will feel. You will feel happiness, anger, sadness, anxiety, etc. This could lead to issues with eating, sleeping, and even interacting with others. My best advice? Allow yourself to feel them. Try to figure out what is bringing these feelings on specifically. It's best to do it in a safe place with those whom you trust and understand what you're going through. Schedule some time where you can allow yourself to dig deep into these feelings. And understand it's okay to not feel OK. Time heals all. You just have to let it.

The idea of closure comes to mind. I personally believe closure is this fictitious wall built on our path to stop us from the temptation of believing it's not done. There's still a chance, right? Well, there's always a chance. The question is, how much is that lottery ticket worth to you? Are you going to go into work every day while being underpaid and underappreciated just because you were promised something that doesn't seem like it's coming? Are you going to wait by the phone for that date to call you back even though a few weeks have passed? There's still a chance, you mutter to yourself as you keep waiting. You feel like you can't abandon it because they never said it's done or over, or they keep promising that it's going to happen for you. You're left in emotional limbo.

My recommendation is, if your requests aren't met in the timeframe you've set and yes, you should set limits on how much you're willing to take and how long you're willing to take it call that your closure. You know you don't deserve to be treated that way. If you continue holding on past your set timeframe, the blame is now on yourself. It may help to create a ritual, something special you do which you normally don't, to signify the end of an endeavor. Think of it as a timer going off to tell you it's done, your way of training yourself to let go.

Remember, it's not failure but progress. If something doesn't meet your requirements, your standards, or your timeframe, then you have every right to walk away. At times it could feel like a failure, but in the grand scheme of things, staying would derail your plans for your bigger picture. Every step you take towards your life goals is progress, but so is avoiding steps that take you away from that.

Let's say you own a small boutique that sells watches. Your watches cost you $100 apiece, and you sell them for $150. A customer comes in only wanting to pay $99. What do you say to that? Are you willing to lose a dollar just because someone asked? Probably not. I mean, that takes away from your goals of being a profitable business. And if you wouldn't do it for your store, why would you do it with your time, energy, and life? It's really no different. Despite how important money is in this world, time is way more valuable. We all do the best we can within our budget. Sometimes we might buy things that we need to return. Has that ever made you feel like a failure? Just the same if you left a job that didn't serve you or a romantic partner that caused more heartache than joy. Always come back to the big picture and let it be your guiding light.

Your time and energy are currency you can't get back. They can only be traded for things. Every promise made to you is a wager that costs time and energy. Sometimes the person you're betting on is trustworthy or has facts to back up their claim. Other times, you're about to be swindled out of as much as they can take from you. And just like gambling, there are some people who will lose everything and there are other people who gamble responsibly, who go in with a set amount they're willing to lose, and if they lose that, they will leave.

What I'm getting at here is if you come up with a plan, a strict set of parameters that must be followed, you will find yourself not falling under the sunk cost fallacy as often. Think of what you want, what you'd like to have, and how long you have to get it. Also, think of the deal breakers that could instantly end this partnership. If your conditions aren't met, walk away. I know it can be tough sometimes, but stick to your guns.

I've probably used more examples than necessary, but this is something I'm quite passionate about.

Time and time again, I see people throwing away their time, energy, and future. If there's any way I could explain it better, I would. The simplest lesson to learn is, when it stops being worthy, you walk away.

WALKING AWAY

There is always a point in our lives where the juice isn't worth the squeeze, or we bark up the wrong tree. A powerful, energy saving, time saving technique must be implemented, also known as walking away.

Admittedly, it sounds simple in theory but proves to be a daunting task in practice, particularly when our emotions are entangled, whether through love or spite. We convince ourselves that persisting is the best course of action, often losing sight of the true cost of our investment. I'm not referring to challenges that appear daunting but hold promise with effort and persistence. I'm addressing dead-end situations where success is virtually impossible, scenarios where even if we were to succeed, the victory would be hollow, serving only to stroke our ego.

Consider these scenarios:

Imagine applying for a job only to discover during the interview that you lack the required credentials. Despite your conviction that you're more than capable, the company simply can't hire you. Yet, you persist, bombarding them with calls and emails, pleading your case. This is wasted effort. The smart move would be to either acquire the necessary credentials or seek similar opportunities elsewhere.

Now, picture yourself trying to rent an apartment. Regardless of your enthusiasm, the landlord has already written you off. Despite your best efforts, it's clear you won't sway their decision. Persisting will only worsen the situation. Move on and search for another place, leaving the door open for reconsideration if their stance changes.

Finally, consider a date that you felt went exceptionally well. Yet, your date doesn't share your sentiment and politely expresses their disinterest. Despite their clear message, you persist, attempting to change their mind until they block you. It's time to walk away gracefully. Continuing to pursue someone who isn't interested is futile and disrespectful. Move forward and find someone who shares your enthusiasm. Besides, why would you want to be with someone who doesn't want to be with you.

In each of these scenarios, continuing the struggle is akin to fighting a lost battle. Investing more time, energy, and emotion will only lead to further frustration and disappointment. Learning to discern between a tough battle and a lost cause is crucial for your well-being. Accepting rejection and moving on is not a sign of weakness but rather a display of maturity and self-respect.

Now, let's delve deeper into why walking away is not only a pragmatic choice but also an empowering one.

- **Preserving Your Resources:** Every action we take requires resources—time, energy, and emotional investment. When we persist in futile endeavors, we drain these finite resources, leaving us depleted and unable to pursue more fruitful opportunities. By recognizing when to walk away, we conserve these resources, allowing us to redirect them towards endeavors with greater potential for success.

- **Maintaining Self-Respect:** Continuously pursuing something or someone who has made it clear they're not interested undermines our self-respect. It communicates a lack of regard for our own worth and boundaries. Walking away on the other hand, demonstrates self-assurance and respect for oneself. It sends a message that we value our time and dignity too much to waste them on fruitless pursuits.

- **Embracing Growth and Adaptation:** Walking away from a dead-end situation isn't just about avoiding further frustration; it's also an opportunity for growth and adaptation. It forces us to reevaluate our goals and strategies, encouraging us to seek alternative paths to success. In doing so, we cultivate resilience and flexibility, essential qualities for navigating life's inevitable challenges and setbacks.

- **Opening Doors to New Opportunities:** Closing the door on one opportunity often opens windows to countless others. When we let go of what isn't right for us, we create space for new possibilities to emerge. Whether it's a career opportunity, a living arrangement, or a relationship, walking away paves the way for fresh beginnings and unexpected blessings.

- **Honoring Personal Boundaries:** Walking away is an act of setting and honoring personal boundaries. It's a declaration that we refuse to tolerate mistreatment, rejection, or neglect. By respecting our boundaries, we command respect from others and create healthier, more fulfilling relationships and experiences.

In essence, walking away is not a sign of defeat but rather a strategic choice, one that prioritizes self-respect, growth, and well-being. It's a declaration of empowerment a refusal to be held captive by futile endeavors or toxic situations. So, the next time you find yourself facing a dead end, remember the power of walking away. In doing so, you reclaim control over your destiny and pave the way for a brighter, more fulfilling future.

SECTION 4
LESSONS TO FOLLOW

KINTSUGI

Transport yourself to 15th-century Japan, where the captivating tale begins. Legend has it that the esteemed shogun Ashikaga Yoshimasa found himself in a predicament when his cherished Chinese tea bowl met an untimely demise, shattered into irreparable fragments. Seeking a solution that would honor both its utility and its intrinsic beauty, Japanese artisans turned to the ancient technique of lacquer work. These skilled craftsmen blended it with powdered gold, silver, or platinum, creating a radiant adhesive that would fill the cracks and crevasses with a luminous embrace. Kintsugi was born not only as a method of repair but a profound philosophy that transcended the material realm.

At its heart lies wabi-sabi, the quintessentially Japanese aesthetic that embraces impermanence and imperfection. In the simplicity of a cracked vessel, the Japanese found a mirror to the momentary nature of existence and the subtle beauty of the flawed. Each fracture became not a mark of shame but a badge of honor, a testament to the object's resilience and enduring spirit.

As the art of kintsugi flourished, it became more than just a practical solution; it evolved into a symbol of renewal and transformation. With every painstaking repair, the artisans infused the ceramic with a new chapter of its story, weaving a tapestry of memories and experiences that made it even more precious than before. Through the centuries, kintsugi endured as a cherished tradition, a timeless reminder of the inherent beauty in imperfection. Its allure lies not only in its exquisite craftsmanship but also in its profound symbolism—a testament to the resilience of the human spirit and the power of embracing life's fractures as part of a greater, more radiant whole.

So, as you behold a kintsugi masterpiece, let yourself be transported to a realm where brokenness is not an end but a beginning, where imperfection is not a flaw but a source of beauty. In that moment of contemplation, may you find solace in the wisdom of the ages—a reminder that our scars do not diminish us but enrich us, and that true beauty lies in the art of embracing life's imperfections with grace and humility.

Think about that for a second. Embracing the cracks. Embracing the repairs. Embracing the history of an object that is one-of-a-kind because of what it has been through. Essentially, we're all born the same, a clean slate, perfect little humans. It's our life that shapes us who we are. We make a mistake, crack, we learn from it, crack fixed. Each and every one of us living a completely different life, even identical twins, live in see life differently. We become products of our environment. Seeing life differently makes similar challenges we face different.

There is no better time in history to be proud, to be an individual, to not hide our cracks, but to embrace them. Share them like a kintsugi bowl for others to admire or learn from or like Wabi Sabi imperfect, impermanent, and incomplete, yet beautiful and unique. So many of us strive for perfection, but funny enough each and every one of us has a different idea of what perfection is. Each and every crack wonders and leads into a different direction. Has a different beginning and a different end.

The moral of the story, we've all been through stuff, and it's exactly that stuff that's made us who we are, that's made us unique for each lesson we've learn, that shapes our very own way of thinking. Some of us may have had a rough time and because of that may even carry anger or shame. Even though it can't be cured overnight, it can be cured. A lesson to learn, a crack being fixed. A reason to let the shame or anger go, and to embrace the experience as a whole, so that it may never happen again. Cracked fixed, fixed so well it will never crack there again.

SOCIAL MEDIA: THE MIRROR YOU DIDN'T KNOW YOU WERE LOOKING INTO

More and more people are expressing discontent with social media, labeling it as fake and toxic. Have you ever found yourself questioning the authenticity of someone's vacation photos or doubting the sincerity behind a friend's posts? These sentiments have become commonplace among social media users, prompting discussions about its true nature and impact on our lives.

Consider the evolution of professional wrestling. Once believed to be a genuine sport, it gradually transformed into entertainment. Fans became aware of the scripted nature of matches and storylines, yet the popularity of wrestling soared. Similarly, reality TV shows present exaggerated versions of reality, captivating millions of viewers with their absurdity. In light of these examples, why do we grant wrestling and reality TV a pass while scrutinizing individuals on social media? Even if their posts are embellished or outright lies, does it truly affect our lives? Perhaps the real question is: why does it bother us?

If we're honest with ourselves, our discomfort often stems from jealousy or comparison. We may resent the attention others receive or covet aspects of their lives. But dwelling on these feelings only reveals our own insecurities and shortcomings. Instead of indulging in envy, we should focus on self-reflection and personal growth. Social media has also been blamed for destroying relationships, but this accusation overlooks individual accountability. Blaming a platform for the actions of its users is misguided. Social media merely amplifies human behavior; it doesn't dictate it. If anything, it exposes the flaws and mistakes we're prone to making, whether it's cheating or succumbing to negativity. Scrolling through social media can evoke a range of emotions, from laughter to anger to empathy. Each reaction offers insight into our true selves, revealing our values, biases, and desires. Rather than passively consuming content, we should actively question our reactions and motivations. By understanding our feelings and their underlying causes, we can cultivate greater self-awareness and resilience.

In essence, social media is a tool—a reflection of humanity's triumphs and shortcomings. Its impact depends on how we choose to wield it. Instead of blaming social media for our discontent, let's harness its potential for connection, self-discovery, and positive change. Just as a hammer can be used to build or destroy, so too can social media be a force for good if we use it wisely.

100 YEARS IN PERSPECTIVE

How much time do you think you have left in your life? For most of you, the answer is more than you realize. You probably have at least half, if not the whole lifetime of someone who lived 100 years ago. Back then, the average life expectancy was between 40 to 60 years. Yet, we often feel like we have no time and life is too short. Why is that?

How has life changed in the past 100 years compared to today?

- **Transportation:** 100 years ago, most people traveled by horse, bicycle, train, or foot. Today, most people have access to cars, buses, subways, trains, and airplanes that can take them anywhere in the world in a matter of hours or days.

- **Communication:** 100 years ago, most people communicated by mail, telegram, radio, or word of mouth. Today, most people have access to the internet, which provides them with unlimited instant information and communication.

- **Education:** 100 years ago, most people had little or no formal education. Today, most people have access to free and compulsory education, and many continue to higher education or vocational training.

- **Entertainment:** 100 years ago, most people had few options for entertainment. Today, most people have access to a wide range of entertainment, from music and movies to sports and games.

- **Shopping:** 100 years ago, most people had to make or grow their own food, clothes, and other necessities. Today, most people have access to supermarkets, malls, online stores, and delivery services that offer a wide range of products at affordable prices.
- **Working:** 100 years ago, most people worked in agriculture, manufacturing, or domestic service. Today, most people work in services, technology, or creative industries.

Life 100 years ago was slower, simpler, and more local; life now is faster, more complex, and more global. Given these changes, we should be grateful for the opportunities and benefits that life now offers us and not take them for granted. We should also be mindful of the challenges and risks that life now poses to us and not ignore them. We should make the most of our time and resources and not waste them. We should also take more time for ourselves, and not neglect our physical, mental, and emotional well-being. We should appreciate the present and not forget the past or the future.

We should also remember that we are never too old to chase our dreams, no matter what they are. Age is not a barrier but a number. Many people have achieved their dreams later in life, proving that it is never too late to pursue your passion just like Samuel L. Jackson, who didn't land his defining role in "Pulp Fiction" until he was 46, or Ray Kroc, who only began building the McDonald's empire when he was in his 50s. Laura Ingalls Wilder published her first "Little House" book when she was 65, and Grandma Moses started painting when she was 76, becoming a famous folk artist. Harland Sanders franchised his Kentucky Fried Chicken business when he was 62.

These individuals, and many others like them, demonstrate that age is not a factor in chasing your dreams. They show that you can achieve anything you set your mind to as long as you have the courage, the persistence, and the belief in yourself. They inspire us to follow our hearts and live our lives to the fullest. Don't let age stop you. You have more time than you think, and you have the potential to make it count. As George Eliot once said, "It is never too late to be what you might have been."

IS HAPPINESS CONTAGIOUS?

Happiness is a powerful emotion that has the potential to spread from one person to another, influencing not only individuals but entire communities. When we experience happiness, it can positively impact those around us, creating a ripple effect that enhances the well-being of others. This concept suggests that our emotions are interconnected, and our happiness can inspire joy and positivity in others.

Consider how you feel when you're around someone who radiates happiness. Their laughter, positive energy, and optimistic outlook can lift your spirits and make you feel better. This phenomenon is not just a coincidence; it's rooted in psychological and social dynamics. When we see others happy, our brains respond in kind, releasing feel-good chemicals like dopamine and serotonin. This response not only improves our mood but also fosters a sense of connection and empathy.

But what happens when the opposite is true? When we're surrounded by negativity or sadness, it can be equally contagious. This is why it's important to be mindful of the company we keep and the environments we spend time in. Just as happiness can spread, so can stress and unhappiness. By choosing to surround ourselves with positive influences, we can create a supportive network that uplifts and motivates us.

It's important to recognize the role we play in this emotional exchange. We have the power to influence others with our attitude and actions. By actively cultivating our own happiness, we can contribute to the well-being of those around us. Simple acts of kindness, gratitude, and positivity can go a long way in creating a harmonious and joyful environment. Moreover, understanding the contagious nature of happiness encourages us to be more compassionate and supportive of others. When we see someone struggling, offering a kind word or a helping hand can make a significant difference in their emotional state. Our empathy and generosity can create a positive feedback loop, where our actions inspire others to spread happiness as well.

In addition to social interactions, the media we consume also plays a role in our emotional well-being. Positive and uplifting content can boost our mood, while negative or distressing news can bring us down. Being selective about what we watch, read, and listen to can help us maintain a more positive outlook on life. It's about finding a balance and being conscious of how external influences affect our internal state.

Practicing mindfulness and self-care is another crucial aspect of maintaining happiness. Taking time to reflect on what brings us joy, setting personal goals, and engaging in activities that nurture our mind and body can enhance our overall sense of well-being. When we prioritize our happiness, we become better equipped to handle life's challenges and share our positive energy with others.

Ultimately, happiness is a shared journey. By recognizing its contagious nature, we can take proactive steps to foster positivity in ourselves and our communities. Each smile, kind gesture, and moment of joy has the potential to create a ripple effect, spreading happiness far and wide. So let's embrace the power of happiness and make a conscious effort to share it with those around us. In doing so, we not only improve our own lives but also contribute to a happier, more connected world.

THE SPOTLIGHT EFFECT

Have you ever found yourself in a situation where you tripped in public or said something embarrassing, feeling like all eyes were on you? It's a universal experience, driven by what psychologists call the spotlight effect—the tendency to overestimate how much attention others pay to us. But what if I told you that most people didn't even notice, let alone care?

The spotlight effect tricks us into believing that everyone is scrutinizing our every move, when in reality, they're just as preoccupied with their own lives and concerns (probably worried about being watched themselves). We hesitate to take risks or pursue our passions out of fear of judgment, forgetting that the opinions of strangers hold little weight in the grand scheme of things.

Consider the last time you had a mishap in public. Maybe you stumbled over your words during a presentation or spilled your coffee on your shirt. In that moment, you might have felt a surge of embarrassment, convinced that all eyes were on you. But truthfully, most people probably didn't even notice, and those who did likely moved on with their day without giving it a second thought.

We are all the protagonists of our own stories, and while we may briefly glance at others, our attention quickly returns to our own lives. Think back to your childhood, when you were carefree and uninhibited. You said and did things without worrying about what others might think. At what point did you start caring about the opinions of others? More importantly, what dreams or aspirations did you abandon because of this concern?

As children, we are fearless in our pursuits, unencumbered by societal expectations. We dance, sing, and create without fear of judgment simply because it brings us joy. But as we grow older, we become more attuned to the opinions of others, often at the expense of our own happiness and fulfillment.

Once Upon a time, there was a little boy named Tommy. Tommy loved to dance and sing. He would dance and sing all the time, including when walking to and from school. Well, one day the neighbors gave Tommy a very weird look while Tommy was dancing and singing his way home from school. He felt embarrassed for the first time. Rather than continuing his song and dance, he stopped immediately never to sing and dance again. Instead, he became an accountant (Not that being an accountant is bad). But now Tommy daydreams of what could have been. Maybe he was the next pop superstar or a professional dancer on Broadway. We will never know. Am I being dramatic, absolutely, but Tommy's story serves as a cautionary tale of the dangers of letting the fear of judgment dictate our actions. By succumbing to the spotlight effect, Tommy denied himself the opportunity to pursue his passions and live life on his own terms. Instead of dancing to the beat of his own drum, he chose the safe path, never daring to dream of what could have been.

So, what's stopping you from stepping out of the spotlight and reclaiming your freedom? Fear, of course, but fear is just an illusion—a barrier we create in our minds. Challenge yourself to do something mildly embarrassing in a place where you rarely go. Record a video of yourself talking about your day or why you've avoided that place. Embrace the discomfort, knowing that the opinions of strangers hold little significance in your life.

Consider this, have you ever noticed someone taking a selfie or recording themselves in public? Did you give it much thought afterward? Probably not. And yet, when it comes to doing the same thing ourselves, we hesitate out of fear of judgment. We worry about how we'll be perceived by strangers, forgetting that their opinions hold little weight in the grand scheme of things. Imagine you're at a party, surrounded by people you don't know very well. You feel self-conscious and awkward, worrying about how others perceive you. But here's the thing: most people are too focused on their own conversations and interactions to pay much attention to you. By reminding yourself of this fact, you can ease your social anxiety and engage more confidently with those around you.

I believe that not letting the opinions of others affect you is a superpower. It's a strength I strive to cultivate every day. That's not to say you should disregard the advice of those who care about you or are more knowledgeable than you. But ultimately, the decision should be yours and yours alone. If someone doesn't understand or support your aspirations, perhaps they don't belong in your inner circle.

Remember, if people are going to watch, you might as well give them a show. Don't let the fear of judgment hold you back from pursuing your passions and dreams. Embrace the spotlight, knowing that it's not as bright or unforgiving as it seems. Step into the light and shine brightly, unencumbered by the opinions of others. Your authenticity and passion will inspire those around you, and you'll pave the way for others to do the same. So go ahead and dance like nobody's watching, because in reality, they're not.

As you reflect on your journey to overcome the spotlight effect, remember that it's a gradual process. Be patient with yourself and celebrate each small victory along the way. By stepping out of the spotlight and embracing your true self, you'll unlock a world of possibilities and live life on your own terms.

DO THE CLOTHES MAKE THE PERSON? OR IS IT THE PERSON WHO MAKES THE CLOTHES LOOK GOOD?

It's a thought-provoking inquiry that has sparked countless debates among philosophers, psychologists, and fashion enthusiasts alike. But let's dive deeper, shall we? Beyond the surface lies a profound truth: our clothing possesses a remarkable ability to shape not only how others perceive us but also how we perceive ourselves.

This reminds me of an amazing memory. It was my nephew's first communion (an important Catholic religious ceremony), and I had custom suits made for him and his younger brother. When they put those suits on, they felt like a million bucks. They both walked so proudly despite their classmates being slightly underdressed in comparison. Other parents showed them attention, complimenting them on their outfits. You could see the confidence dripping out of them. They felt completely seen. They weren't just a couple of kids; they were transformed into more mature youths.

Think back to the days of your childhood when the world was a playground and your imagination knew no bounds. Remember the sheer joy of playing dress-up, transforming into superheroes, princesses, or intrepid explorers with just a few pieces of fabric? In those magical moments, our clothing wasn't just fabric; it was a portal to adventure, allowing us to step into new roles and learn valuable lessons about bravery, creativity, and self-expression.

Adolescence—the rollercoaster ride of self-discovery and identity formation. During those formative years, our clothing becomes more than just a means of covering our bodies; it becomes a tool for self-expression and exploration. We eagerly emulate our role models, whether they be our parents, favorite celebrities, or fictional characters, through our fashion choices. With each outfit, we assert our individuality and stake our claim in the world, yearning to be seen, understood, and accepted for who we truly are.

As we transition into adulthood, our relationship with clothing continues to evolve, mirroring our growing sense of self-awareness and confidence. Whether we're dressing for a job interview, a first date, or a night out with friends, our attire speaks volumes about who we are and what we value. Just like my nephews in their suits, we experience a surge in self-esteem when we take the time to present ourselves with care and attention to detail.

At its core, the act of dressing ourselves is an act of self-care and self-expression. When we put effort into our appearance, we're sending a powerful message to ourselves and the world: "I am worthy of love, attention, and respect." Just as we invest time and energy into maintaining our physical health through exercise and nutrition, so too should we prioritize our sartorial well-being as a vital component of our overall wellness. Remember, the opposite has a similar effect. It can make us feel down, lethargic, and self-loathing. I'm sure I've said this multiple times already, the way we treat ourselves is the way we accept others to treat us. Not to mention it becomes infinitely harder to accept compliments as we don't believe someone could see us any differently.

Now, let's talk personal style. It's not just about following the latest trends or conforming to societal expectations; it's about expressing who you are and what you stand for. Whether you gravitate towards classic elegance, edgy experimentation, or bohemian whimsy, your clothing is a canvas upon which you can paint your unique essence. In every country, in every state or province, every city, every genre of music, every hobby, etc. Style is different, especially in the time we live in now more than ever. So you might as well wear whatever makes you happy. Our relationship with clothing goes beyond the physical; it is deeply intertwined with our emotions and memories. Think about your favorite piece of clothing—the one that holds sentimental value or evokes a rush of nostalgia. Maybe it's your grandmother's vintage dress or the jacket you wore on your first date. These garments carry with them a piece of our history, reminding us of cherished moments and the people we hold dear.

Life is a series of transitions, each marked by its own sartorial significance. Whether you're starting a new job, moving to a new city, or embarking on a new relationship, your clothing can serve as a source of comfort and confidence during times of change. By dressing with intention and authenticity, you signal to yourself and others that you are ready to embrace whatever the future holds.

Personal style is not static; it evolves and matures alongside us, reflecting our growth and experiences. What resonated with us in our youth may no longer align with our current selves, and that's perfectly okay. Embracing the evolution of our style allows us to embrace change with open arms and embark on new style journeys with enthusiasm and curiosity.

Incorporating rituals into your dressing routine can elevate the experience from mundane to meaningful. Whether it's taking a few moments to appreciate yourself in the mirror or reciting affirmations as you get dressed, these small acts of self-care can have a profound impact on your confidence and self-esteem.

The relationship between clothing and self-esteem is a complex and multifaceted one, encompassing elements of identity, expression, and empowerment. Our wardrobe choices have the power to shape not only how we are perceived by others but also how we perceive ourselves. By embracing the transformative potential of our clothing, we can harness its power to cultivate confidence, foster self-expression, and embark on a journey of self-discovery.

So the next time you reach into your closet, remember: the clothes may indeed make the person, but it is the person who infuses them with meaning, purpose, and undeniable style.

SECTION 5
PERSONAL REFLECTION

YOU NEVER LEARN ANYTHING ON A GOOD DAY

Imagine for a moment a sunny day, with a gentle breeze whispering through the air, and birds singing harmoniously in the background. It's the kind of day where everything seems to fall perfectly into place. You excel in your tasks effortlessly, receiving accolades and admiration from peers and superiors alike. In these moments, it's easy to believe that success is a testament solely to our abilities and talents. Yet, beneath the surface of triumph lies a subtle deception. Success, in its pristine form, often masks the valuable lessons that can only be gathered from failure. When everything goes according to plan, there's little incentive to question our methods or seek alternative paths. We become complacent, lulled into a false sense of security by the illusion of our infallibility. The danger of such complacency is that it blinds us to the reality of our limitations. We begin to believe that success is our birthright, rather than the result of hard work, perseverance, and a willingness to embrace failure. In doing so, we rob ourselves of the opportunity to grow and evolve, trapped in a cycle of stagnation and mediocrity.

Contrary to popular belief, mistakes are not the opposite of success; rather, they are its essential counterpart. Consider the story of Thomas Edison, whose relentless pursuit of the electric light bulb was riddled with countless failures. Each setback, far from deterring him, served as a stepping stone towards his ultimate triumph. When asked about his repeated failures, Edison famously remarked, "I have not failed. I've just found 10,000 ways that won't work."

Similarly, in our own lives, it's crucial to reframe our perspective on mistakes. Instead of viewing them as indicators of inadequacy, we should embrace them as opportunities for growth and self-discovery. Every misstep, every blunder, holds within it a valuable lesson waiting to be unearthed. By acknowledging our shortcoming, we open ourselves up to a wealth of knowledge and experience that would otherwise remain inaccessible.

Even on good days, when success comes easy, it's important to be mindful of our achievements. It's easy to take success for granted when everything falls into place effortlessly. But by being mindful of our successes, we can appreciate the hard work and effort that went into achieving them. It's about acknowledging the role of luck and circumstance, rather than attributing success solely to our abilities. Mindfulness isn't just about being present in moments of struggle; it's also about being present in moments of success. It's about savoring the victories, no matter how small, acknowledging the effort that went into achieving them, and the countless failures that lead us here. By being mindful of our successes, we cultivate gratitude and humility, recognizing that success is not guaranteed and should never be taken for granted.

Learning from our mistakes is not a passive process but rather an active endeavor fueled by reflection and introspection. It requires us to confront our shortcomings with honesty and humility, to dissect the root causes of our failures, and to extract valuable insights for the future. By cultivating a mindset of continuous learning, we transform our setbacks into springboards for personal and professional development.

Resilience is the bedrock upon which we build our capacity to weather life's storms and emerge stronger on the other side. It is the willingness to embrace failure as an integral part of the human experience, recognizing that adversity is not a barrier but a catalyst for growth. By reframing our perception of setbacks, we empower ourselves to confront challenges with courage and resilience.

Consider the analogy of a phoenix rising from the ashes—a symbol of resilience and renewal in the face of adversity. Like the mythical bird, we possess an innate ability to transcend our limitations and soar to new heights. It is through our struggles and hardships that we discover the depths of our resilience, forging a path towards personal mastery and fulfillment.

In the journey of life, success and failure are not mutually exclusive but rather two sides of the same coin. It is through our mistakes that we gain the wisdom to navigate the complexities of the human experience, forging a path towards self-discovery and growth. By embracing our imperfections with courage and resilience, we unlock the transformative power of learning and emerge as architects of our own destiny. Remember, you never learn anything on a good day. It is in the test of adversity that true learning takes place, shaping us into the best versions of ourselves. So, the next time you find yourself confronted by failure, embrace it as an opportunity for growth, knowing that within every setback lies the seed of triumph. And when you are blessed with easy success, be mindful of how it came to be and grateful it happened in the first place.

As the Chinese proverb wisely states, "Failure is not falling down but refusing to get up." Embrace your mistakes, learn from them, and let them propel you towards greatness.

AGE VS EXPERIENCE

A common theme in this book is being honest with yourself. The importance of being able to realize you might not know something you thought you did. Age versus experience is a perfect example. Let me ask you this. When did you learn to do your laundry? Me personally, I was eight or nine, I think. I'll ask my mom to be sure. Some of us learned at a young age, while some may still not know how to do it. I'm sure there are college kids all over the world messing up their first load of laundry. Just because you're an adult and have watched mom or dad do it doesn't mean you know how. Then again, with the invention of YouTube, I'm sure less mistakes are being made.

Here's a story about something a little more complex. So, as I'm writing this book, I met a woman. For the sake of this story, let's call her Sam. Sam was turning 40, had been separated from her toxic husband for the past two years, and was just starting to get her feet wet in the dating scene. It almost sounds normal for this day and age, but this was technically her first time dating as she's been with her husband since she was a teenager. Imagine that, never slept with anyone else, never ghosted or was ghosted, never played the stupid games people play with each other when dating, etc.

So, as I got to know her on a more personal level, I felt it was my duty to give her a little crash course in dating (Revised for 2023). To be honest, it didn't go so well. Apparently, she knew everything already. Specifically told me she knew the games guys played and she doesn't play these games or tolerate it. She knew what ghosting was and didn't care. She was emotionally ready to handle the dating world. She sounded surer of herself than a teenage boy about to drive for the first time. Was she right? Did she know what she was doing? No, of course not.

She started to get to know a guy. As far as she told me, he would pressure her to see her daily as he lived not too far away. He talked to her all throughout the day showering her with attention, which she loved. But that all came to an end after they slept together about six days after meeting. All of a sudden, he seemed busy and distant, no time to meet her anymore. Even when she expressed her feelings, his rebuttal would be that she was delusional. She would get so angry with him that she would ignore his texts (even though they were far and few between). She confessed to me that this was messing up her life. She couldn't get over him even though she was trying to. She took none of my recommendations and ended up very troubled. I don't know what happened to her, as I can't help those who don't help themselves. We eventually lost touch.

That story displays what could happen if we aren't honest with ourselves, even with me explaining that her lack of experience could get her into trouble, and apparently her best friends warned her as well. Just because she was 40, that doesn't mean she knew how to date (granted a little more complicated than laundry). I hope she got over it and moved on in a positive direction. There are instances where presuming we know something could be more dangerous than not knowing it at all, it could even end up in physical harm or worse.

Here is another example.

In the bustling office of Tech Innovations, a scene of quiet respect unfolds each day. At the helm is Julian, a manager whose youthful appearance often prompts a second glance. He's significantly younger than his team, yet his chair at the head of the conference table is no accident. Julian's ascent to management was not a product of time served but of knowledge earned.

His team, seasoned professionals with years of experience, initially met Julian's appointment with skepticism. However, it wasn't long before they recognized the wisdom behind the decision. Julian had a knack for technology that seemed almost intuitive. He could predict market trends with uncanny accuracy and had a portfolio of successful projects that opposed his age. Under his guidance, the team flourished, achieving milestones that had previously seemed out of reach. His innovative strategies and fresh perspectives breathed new life into projects that had stalled under conventional approaches. Julian's age became an afterthought, overshadowed by the results he consistently delivered. The employees, once wary, now seek Julian's counsel on critical decisions. They value his expertise, which has propelled the company forward and, in turn, advanced their own careers. In the world of Tech Innovations, it's clear that experience isn't just measured in years; it's measured in achievements. And in that regard, Julian stands tall among his peers.

This story demonstrates how a young person with the right experience and knowledge can be better suited for a position than someone older with more experience. It highlights the importance of skill and performance over age in professional settings.

The tug-of-war between age and experience highlights a crucial lesson: staying honest with oneself is key. The stories shared shed light on the stark outcomes of assuming knowledge versus acknowledging one's limits.

Take the case of Sam, for instance. Her journey serves as a cautionary tale on the dangers of thinking you know it all. Despite her age, well-meaning advice, and warnings, her lack of dating experience led her down a rocky path, causing emotional turmoil. It's a stark reminder that staying humble and open to learning is vital, no matter your age or situation.

Julian's story paints a picture of how skill and insight can trump age. Leading the pack at Tech Innovations, Julian proves that it's not about how long you've been around, but what you bring to the table. His knack for technology and strategic thinking propelled him to the top, earning him the respect of his older peers.

In essence, whether navigating the complexities of personal relationships or excelling in the professional arena, the moral remains crystal clear: staying true to yourself, knowing your limitations, and embracing a mindset of continuous growth are the keys to triumph, regardless of your age.

GOOD HEALTH IS INDEED A CROWN ON A WELL PERSON'S HEAD

"One that often goes unnoticed until it's lost"

By recognizing the importance of our health and taking proactive steps to nurture it, we not only safeguard our physical well-being but also enhance our mental and emotional resilience. Every small effort towards improving our health matters, as each positive choice contributes to the bigger picture of our overall well-being.

In today's fast-paced world, it's all too easy to take our health for granted. With hectic schedules, demanding workloads, and endless distractions, our well-being often takes a backseat. We may find ourselves reaching for convenience foods, skipping workouts, and sacrificing sleep in the pursuit of productivity. But what we fail to realize is that neglecting our health today can have serious consequences tomorrow.

Consider for instance, the impact of chronic stress on our bodies. When we're constantly under pressure, our bodies release cortisol, a hormone that can wreak havoc on our physical and mental health. Chronic stress has been linked to a host of health problems, including heart disease, diabetes, and depression. By prioritizing our health and finding ways to manage stress effectively, we can reduce our risk of these serious conditions and lead happier, more fulfilling lives.

Moreover, the benefits of good health extend far beyond the physical realm. When our bodies are in good shape, our minds tend to follow suit. We feel more alert, focused, and mentally resilient. The energy and vitality gained from a healthy lifestyle can enhance our mood, boost our self-confidence, and improve our overall quality of life. On the other hand, neglecting our health can lead to feelings of lethargy, irritability, and low self-esteem. By investing in our health, we not only improve our physical well-being but also cultivate a positive mindset that empowers us to tackle life's challenges with confidence and resilience.

But how do we go about prioritizing our health in a world filled with competing demands and distractions? The key lies in making conscious choices that support our well-being, one step at a time. It's not about making drastic changes overnight or adhering to strict diet and exercise regimens. Instead, it's about finding sustainable practices that work for us and integrating them into our daily lives. If what we do isn't sustainable, there will be no chance that we could be consistent. That is the reason why most diets don't work and gym memberships don't get used. Every small effort towards improving our health matters, whether it's choosing a salad over a burger, taking the stairs instead of the elevator, or committing to a short daily walk.

These seemingly insignificant choices may not yield immediate results, but over time, they add up to significant improvements in our overall well-being. They are also easy enough choices to be sustainable and consistent. By focusing on our progress we can gradually build healthier habits that become ingrained in our daily routines. Of course, prioritizing our health isn't always easy. It requires discipline, commitment, and at times a willingness to step outside our comfort zones. There will be days when we'd rather hit the snooze button than lace up our running shoes, or reach for the cookie jar instead of the fruit bowl. But it's during these moments of temptation that our resolve is truly tested.

By staying mindful of our goals and reminding ourselves of the benefits of good health, we can overcome these obstacles and stay on track towards achieving our wellness objectives.

It's also important to recognize that prioritizing our health is a journey, not a destination. There will be ups and downs along the way, and setbacks are inevitable. But what matters most is our willingness to keep moving forward, one step at a time. By embracing the process and staying committed to our goals, we can create lasting change that positively impacts every aspect of our lives.

Prioritizing our health is one of the most important investments we can make in ourselves. By recognizing the importance of our well-being and taking proactive steps to nurture it, we can enjoy happier, more fulfilling lives. Every small effort towards improving our health matters, and by making conscious choices that support our well-being, we can create a brighter future for ourselves and those we care about. So let's commit to prioritizing our health today, knowing that the benefits will last a lifetime.

WORRYING DOES NOT TAKE AWAY TOMORROW'S TROUBLES; IT TAKES AWAY TODAY'S PEACE.

Before reading on, take a second and think about all the things you're worried about. Now, out of all those things, how many are an actual priority? I'm sure you've realized most of it isn't all that important.

Why?

Honestly, that all depends on you as a person. Do you let the world's issues get to you or are you focused more on your own life. Do you overextend yourself worrying about other people's problems because you're extremely compassionate? Maybe you shouldn't. I'm not saying you shouldn't give a voice to those issues you believe in but there is something to be said about your own mental health and wellbeing. Not to mention if these existential crises are affecting your daily life, it may be time to discover your inner peace.

We devote time and energy spent in our own thoughts going through any and every scenario, figuring out the best course of action in a situation to solve it or incur the least amount of damage possible.

In a lot of situations, I would champion overthinking, but to a point. It's great to be prepared, but knowing where that point is to where we must just let go and trust our own abilities is vital. Most things aren't worth losing sleep over and it's not like you can do much while you're sleeping anyway. Besides, being well rested will trump overthinking nine times out of ten. Even if you were able to go through every possible situation in your head. I'm sure you'd forget one, the one that happens. Ask yourself (actually ask yourself) is it worth the lack of sleep and anxiety? Is it worth going about your day like a zombie? Potentially forgetting to do something, or too tired to think on your toes. Which leads to more anxiety because you overthink those interactions and situations on how you could have done them differently. And down the spiral we go.

What's worth focusing on is prioritizing your worries from most important to least. As much as I don't think this should be said, I'm going to say it anyway. Your survival is key, as well as your wellbeing (you can't help if you're dead).

How many of your worries do you have direct control over the outcome? At the end of the day, if you're worried about something that you have no control over, how would you be able to be ready to respond? The outcome is based on someone or something else happening. The possibilities of how it will go are endless. Rather, trust yourself that whatever it is you will be able to get through it when the time comes.

Knowing yourself is extremely important. If you know your own abilities, you will be able to deduce if you'll be able to handle a situation regardless of the variables. If you know you can handle a situation, you must not need to worry. More importantly, acknowledge that you'll do your best. It may not help you get your desired outcome, but at least you know how far you can go. A car that runs out of gas can't go any further. It is much easier to come to terms with an undesirable outcome if you know there was nothing else you could have done. And that's okay, moving on is important. You can't win them all, but you can accept it, learn from it, and move forward from it. Speaking of moving forward, leave the past in the past. Unless there is something to be learned, there really is no point in dwelling on it.

I get it, a lot of what I say is easier said than done (in fact most of this book is). It is going to take work on your part to make it happen. In this case, take the time to address every one of your concerns with yourself. Even if that means you schedule time every day or week or month (Depending on the severity).

Train yourself that it is at that time you address things and not at any other time. Figure out the severity, should you be worried or not worry at all. And if you can't seem to get them out of your head, write them down (another common theme). Write them down as soon as those thoughts enter your mind, for you to address later. Use logic and common sense, along with what has happened before in similar situations. The goal here is to keep your mind burden free. To allow yourself to be at peace even if it's for most of the day. Make it a routine, the longer you do it for, the easier it becomes.

SECTION 6
WISDOM

THE THREE-SECOND RULE

How many times have you talked yourself out of trying something in your life? Maybe it was approaching that cute girl or boy standing in the distance. Or perhaps it was deciding on buying those shoes you've been eyeing, only to hesitate long enough that they were sold out. Or maybe it was that job offer you received, but you doubted whether you were capable enough to handle it. Whatever the situation, you thought too long and ended up missing out. Were you lacking confidence in yourself? Worried about what others might think or say? Or maybe it was simply a fear of rejection?

In my youth, I experienced all these feelings. I was small, skinny, and extremely shy. Believe it or not, I was the quiet type. Like most young pre-teens, I just wanted to fit in. When I entered high school, I may have grown physically, but I still could be lost in the crowd. It wasn't until I started hanging out with older kids that I was pushed out of my shell. We used to skip school and hang out at malls or other high schools. Being the youngest and without a car or license, I found myself in an undesirable position. My older friends would force me to approach girls, or else I'd have to find my own way home. Calling for help was out of the question, as my parents would've been furious if they found out. So, what was I to do?

With each passing cute girl, I would count to three and take a step forward. Then another step, and another. Before I knew it, I'd be standing in front of a cute girl with nothing to say. Talk about performing under pressure! But in that moment, I had no choice but to try, because the alternative was impending doom. And so, with my squeaky voice, I would muster up a feeble "Hey" or "Hello." Surprisingly, it worked. After a short conversation, I'd have her number. But my friends were never satisfied; they always demanded more. They wanted me to get 5 phone numbers, then 10, by the end of the school year I ended up with a phone book full of cute girls' numbers. Needless to say, the following summer was a busy one.

Despite what it might seem like, I was rejected more times than I succeeded. But I learned to brush it off and continue with my mission. Failure meant facing my own consequences, but I soldiered on without dwelling on it. You may not have impending danger hanging over your head like I did, but think about it: a lifetime of regret is a real possibility. Regret can haunt you forever. Not taking that leap of faith could leave a bitter taste in your mouth for years to come. Even armed with this knowledge, you might still hesitate, thinking it's a one-in-a-hundred chance. But if I offered you a 100 M&M's, warning that one of them might be deadly, would you still eat them? Probably not. If you think your chances of getting a poisonous M&M is possible, then so is succeeding. So why not take the chance instead of overthinking? Count to three and take a step, then another, until you're right in front of your challenge.

A word of caution: this isn't about recklessness or making life-altering decisions without careful consideration. Just a simple exercise to get yourself more comfortable with being uncomfortable. Learning to pursue what you want when you want it without hesitation. Recognize opportunities in front of you and understand that sometimes, they're worth seizing.

After that year of school, my shyness was mostly gone. But even now, there are times when I have to count to three to get myself moving. Like anyone else, I still fear rejection. But with every rejection, the success feels even sweeter. Now, let's delve deeper into this concept of the Three-Second Rule by exploring a variety of situations where it can be applied:

Imagine yourself at a networking event filled with professionals from your industry. You spot someone you admire or someone who could potentially help you advance in your career. Instead of hesitating and overthinking, employ the Three-Second Rule. Count to three, take a deep breath, and approach them with confidence. Introduce yourself and express your interest in their work or expertise. You'll be surprised how many meaningful connections you can make by simply taking that initial step.

Public speaking can be terrifying for many people. Whether it's giving a presentation at work or speaking at a social gathering, the fear of judgment and failure can hold you back. But with the Three-Second Rule, you can overcome this fear. When it's your turn to speak, don't dwell on your nerves or doubts. Instead, count to three and dive right in. Once you start speaking, you'll find that your confidence grows, and you're able to deliver your message effectively.

Stepping out of your comfort zone often involves trying new activities or hobbies. Whether it's learning a musical instrument, taking up a new sport, or joining a dance class, the fear of failure can be daunting. But by applying the Three-Second Rule, you can overcome this fear and embrace new experiences. Instead of hesitating and making excuses, count to three and take the first step towards trying something new. You'll never know what you're capable of until you try.

Many people struggle with asking for help when they need it. Whether it's seeking guidance on a project at work or asking for support during a difficult time. Pride or fear of rejection can often get in the way. But with the Three-Second Rule, you can overcome this barrier. When you find yourself in need of assistance, don't hesitate to reach out. Count to three and ask for help. You'll be surprised by how willing people are to lend a hand when you're open and vulnerable.

The Three-Second Rule is a powerful tool for overcoming fear, doubt, and hesitation in various aspects of life. By counting to three and taking action, you can push past your comfort zone, seize opportunities, and achieve your goals. So the next time you find yourself hesitating or second-guessing, remember to apply the Three-Second Rule and take that leap of faith. Your future self will thank you for it.

THE POWER OF ACCOMMODATION

In the complexities of human relationships, compromise has often been hailed as the cornerstone of harmony. It's seen as a bridge over troubled waters, the glue that binds different perspectives, a way to make both parties whole. But what if I told you there's a more elegant, more fulfilling approach? What if instead of settling for less, you could aim for more? This is where accommodation steps in, offering a path to not just resolution, but genuine growth and satisfaction.

To truly understand the essence of accommodation, let's first dissect its counterpart: compromise. Compromise, in its simplest form, is the act of meeting halfway. It's finding a middle ground where both parties make concessions, relinquishing certain desires or values to reach a mutually agreeable outcome. While compromise can be effective in resolving conflicts, it often carries an underlying sense of sacrifice. It's akin to splitting the difference, leaving each party with a diluted version of their original intent. Essentially, if we both lose something, it's fair.

Now, contrast that with accommodation. Accommodation goes beyond mere compromise. It involves a profound shift in perspective—a willingness to embrace differences rather than merely reconcile them. Unlike compromise, which may leave both parties feeling like they've lost something, accommodation fosters a sense of empowerment and enrichment for all involved. At its core, accommodation is about adapting and adjusting without sacrificing one's principles or authenticity.

Imagine a scenario where two siblings, Sarah and Alex, are tasked with organizing their parents' anniversary celebration. Sarah is an extrovert who loves large gatherings with music and dancing, while Alex is an introvert who prefers intimate dinners with close family and friends.

In a compromise, Sarah and Alex might agree to host a medium-sized gathering with a live band for a couple of hours, followed by a quieter dinner. While this compromise may seem fair, Sarah may feel disappointed that the party isn't as big and lively as she envisioned, and Alex may feel overwhelmed by the noise and crowds during the band's performance.

Now, let's explore how accommodation could lead to a more satisfying outcome. Instead of settling for a compromise that leaves both sibling feeling slightly unsatisfied, Sarah and Alex choose to accommodate each other's preferences. They sit down for a heartfelt conversation, where Sarah explains how important it is for her to celebrate their parents' milestone with a big, joyous party, while

Alex expresses his desire for a more intimate and relaxed gathering where everyone can truly connect.

With a deeper understanding of each other's perspectives, Sarah and Alex brainstorm creative solutions that accommodate both their preferences. They decide to host a two-part celebration: an early evening dinner at a small restaurant with just immediate family and a few close friends for Alex. Followed by a party with music and dancing for Sarah. By accommodating each other's preferences and planning separate events that cater to their unique tastes, Sarah and Alex create a celebration that is truly meaningful and enjoyable for everyone involved. Sarah gets to dance the night away surrounded by loved ones, while Alex enjoys a cozy evening filled with heartfelt conversations and cherished memories.

This example vividly illustrates the difference between compromise and accommodation. While compromise may involve finding a middle ground between competing interests, accommodation involves actively incorporating each person's desires and preferences into a solution that honors both. In this way, accommodation fosters understanding, cooperation, and ultimately, a more fulfilling experience for everyone involved.

But accommodation isn't just reserved for interpersonal relationships—it's a mindset that can be applied to all aspects of life. Whether we're navigating professional challenges, familial dynamics, or societal conflicts, accommodation invites us to see beyond the surface-level differences and seek common ground rooted in shared values and aspirations.

In the workplace, for instance, accommodation can foster innovation and collaboration by encouraging diverse perspectives and ideas. Instead of enforcing a rigid hierarchy or imposing a one-size-fits-all solution, effective leaders embrace accommodation, recognizing that true success lies in harnessing the collective wisdom and creativity of their team members.

Similarly, on a societal level, accommodation paves the way for progress and social cohesion. By acknowledging and respecting the diverse backgrounds and experiences of individuals within a community, we can create inclusive environments where everyone feels valued and empowered to contribute their unique gifts to the collective good. In essence, accommodation isn't just about finding common ground—it's about cultivating a culture of mutual respect, empathy, and understanding. It's about recognizing that true harmony arises not from erasing differences, but from celebrating them and finding innovative ways to weave them together into the rich tapestry of human experience.

As we embark on this journey of self-discovery and growth, let us embrace the transformative power of accommodation. Let us dare to dream bigger, reach higher, and forge connections that transcend the limitations of compromise. For in the boundless expanse of accommodation, we discover not only the beauty of unity but also the infinite potential of our shared humanity.

THE OXYGEN MASK THEORY

If you've ever traveled by airplane, you're likely familiar with the pre-flight safety instructions. Sitting in your seat, you listen as the flight attendants explain the safety procedures, including what to do in case of an emergency. One key instruction stands out: in the event of a loss of cabin pressure, oxygen masks will drop from the overhead compartments. But here's the crucial part: you must secure your own mask before assisting others.

This simple yet profound instruction holds a valuable life lesson: take care of yourself first before helping others. It's not about selfishness but rather about ensuring that you have the capacity to support others effectively. Just as you can't help others if you're incapacitated, you can't fully support those around you if you neglect your own well-being.

Think back to a time when you were upset or stressed. Did it affect your interactions with others? Did it impact your decision-making ability? Chances are, it did. Our emotional state significantly influences how we engage with the world around us. On the other hand, when we're content and fulfilled, we're better equipped to handle challenges, think clearly, and offer support to others.

For many who have a natural inclination to help others, it can be challenging to prioritize self-care.

There's often a sense of guilt or obligation that arises when we prioritize our own needs. However, neglecting self-care ultimately diminishes our ability to be there for others in the long run.

So, how can we cultivate a practice of prioritizing self-care? Here are a few ideas:

1. **Establish a schedule and routine:** Carve out dedicated time each day for activities that nurture your well-being. Whether it's exercise, meditation, simply enjoying a hobby, prioritizing self-care sends a powerful message that your time and well-being are important.

2. **Practice self-reflection**: Set aside a few minutes each day to reflect on your experiences, emotions, and actions. This practice fosters self-awareness and emotional well-being, helping you identify areas for growth and improvement.

3. **Focus on physical health:** Take care of your body by prioritizing exercise, nutrition, and sleep. Small lifestyle changes, such as choosing healthier food options or getting enough sleep, can have a significant impact on your overall well-being.

4. **Speak to yourself with kindness:** Be mindful of the way you speak to yourself and cultivate a compassionate inner dialogue. Replace negative self-talk with affirming statements that build confidence and self-esteem.

5. **Take pride in yourself:** Treat yourself with the same care and attention you would give to others. Celebrate your achievements, dress in a way that makes you feel good, and practice gratitude for the person you are.

6. **Practice gratitude:** Take time to acknowledge and appreciate the blessings in your life, big and small. Keeping a gratitude journal can be a powerful tool for cultivating a positive outlook and reducing stress.

By actively prioritizing self-care, we not only enhance our own well-being but also increase our capacity to support and uplift those around us. It's a practice that requires intention and commitment, but the rewards greater resilience, fulfillment, and the ability to make a positive impact are well worth the effort. So, remember to secure your own oxygen mask first, and then you'll be better equipped to assist others on life's journey.

SAYING YOU CAN'T, IS SAYING YOU WON'T EVEN TRY

In a world often clouded by negativity, it's easy to lose sight of the immense potential and goodness that surrounds us. From the relentless stream of bad news to our own inner dialogue, negativity has a profound impact on every aspect of our lives. It dampens our spirits, clouds our judgment, and erodes our self-worth, leaving us feeling disillusioned and unfulfilled. But amidst the darkness, there lies a glimmer of hope, a choice to shift our perspective, harness the power of positivity, and embrace a life filled with purpose and fulfillment.

Overcoming Negativity: The Journey Begins Within

The journey to overcome negativity begins with a simple yet profound realization: the words we speak to ourselves hold immense power. Often, without even realizing it, we undermine our own potential and self-worth with a barrage of negative self-talk. We tell ourselves we're not good enough, smart enough, or worthy enough. We dwell on our mistakes, compare ourselves to others, and dismiss our own accomplishments. But this self-criticism is not only unproductive it's detrimental to our well-being.

Empowering Self-Talk: Choosing Positivity

The first step in breaking free from the cycle of negativity is to consciously choose positivity in our self-talk. Instead of berating ourselves for our shortcomings, we must embrace affirmations that uplift and empower us. By affirming our inherent worth, acknowledging our strengths, and celebrating our progress, we reframe our reality and cultivate a mindset of resilience and self-assurance. Through daily repetition and unwavering belief, these positive affirmations become the foundation upon which we build our self-esteem and confidence.

Seeking Constructive Feedback: Navigating the Waters of Criticism

While self-affirmation is crucial, so is the ability to seek feedback and advice from others. However, not all feedback is created equal. In our quest for growth and self-improvement, we must discern between constructive criticism and baseless negativity. When faced with criticism, it's essential to approach it with an open mind and a willingness to learn. By asking probing questions, understanding the perspective of the critic, and extracting value from their insights, we transform criticism into an opportunity for growth. Yet, we must also recognize when criticism lacks merit and learn to trust our own judgment and intuition.

Embracing Action: The Gateway to Self-Discovery

Amidst the sea of uncertainties and doubts, the most effective way to ascertain your capabilities is through action itself. Release the shackles of fear and skepticism and immerse yourself fully in the pursuit of your goals. Disregard the whispers of doubt and the echoes of negativity and focus solely on the exhilarating journey of learning and growth. Through action, you unveil your true potential, shattering the barriers of self-doubt and uncovering hidden reservoirs of resilience and determination. Even in the face of failure, every endeavor yields invaluable lessons and experiences that fortify your spirit and propel you toward greater heights of achievement and self-actualization.

Cultivating Patience: Nurturing the Seeds of Growth

Patience, an invaluable virtue, serves as a guiding beacon amidst the ebb and flow of life's challenges and uncertainties. Recognize that every endeavor requires time and dedication to flourish, much like the gradual mastery of fundamental skills such as walking or language acquisition. In a world conditioned by the allure of instant gratification, embrace the beauty of patience as a steadfast companion on your journey of growth and self-discovery. Celebrate each step forward, no matter how small, and embrace the transformative power of resilience and perseverance in overcoming obstacles and setbacks along the way.

Extending Support: Empowering Others and Ourselves

In our collective journey toward growth and fulfillment, the power of support serves as a beacon of light, illuminating the path for both ourselves and others. Extend a helping hand to those navigating the trials and tribulations of their own pursuits, offering guidance, encouragement, and assistance with compassion and empathy. Through acts of kindness and support, not only do we uplift the spirits of others, but we also foster a culture of collaboration and camaraderie that enriches our own lives. Remember, in all human connections, every gesture of support reverberates with the potential to inspire, uplift, and transform lives.

Navigating the Path Ahead: Embracing Challenges with Resilience and Determination

As we traverse the ever-changing landscape of life, we encounter an array of challenges, setbacks, and uncertainties that test the limits of our resolve and determination. Yet, it is through these adversities that we cultivate the seeds of resilience, fortitude, and unwavering faith in our abilities. Embrace the inevitable trials and tribulations as opportunities for growth and self-discovery, knowing that every obstacle conquered and every setback overcome propels you closer to the realization of your dreams and aspirations. With unwavering faith, determination, and resilience, you possess the power to transcend obstacles, defy expectations, and forge a path of unparalleled success and fulfillment. In the pursuit of our passions and interests, the journey of learning and exploration unfolds as a thrilling adventure—one filled with excitement, discovery, and endless possibilities. If a particular interest or curiosity sparks within you, embrace it wholeheartedly without fear or hesitation. Dive into the depths of research, immerse yourself in educational content, seek guidance from experts, and unravel the intricacies of your chosen pursuit. As you delve deeper into the realm of knowledge, you equip yourself with invaluable insights, skills, and perspectives that enhance your confidence and readiness for the journey ahead. Remember, curiosity is the spark that ignites the flames of creativity and motivation, propelling you toward new horizons of growth and fulfillment.

THE SCORPION AND THE FROG: A PARABLE OF NATURE AND TRUST

A scorpion lived in a dark and dreary cave, longing for a change of scenery. One day, he ventured out and discovered a beautiful land full of greenery and flowers on the other side of a wide river. However, he faced a problem: he couldn't swim, and there was no bridge in sight. As he walked along the riverbank, hoping to find a way across, he spotted a frog sitting on a rock near the water. The scorpion thought, "Maybe that frog can carry me over."

He approached the frog and said, "Hello, friend. I need your help. Could you please swim me across the river?" Startled by the scorpion's request, the frog jumped back and said, "Are you kidding me? Scorpions are known to kill frogs. I'm not going to risk my life for you."

The scorpion replied, "No, no, you have me all wrong. I mean you no harm. I just want to see the other side of the river. If I stung you, we would both drown. I can't swim, you see. I promise I won't hurt you. Please let me ride on your back. It would be a great way to start our friendship."

Intrigued by the scorpion's offer, the frog thought it might be nice to have a scorpion as a friend. He said, "Okay, scorpion, I'll do it. Hop on." The scorpion climbed onto the frog's back, and the frog leaped into the river, swimming towards the opposite shore. Halfway across, the scorpion felt a sudden urge. He raised his tail and stung the frog. The frog felt a sharp pain and numbness spreading through his body. They both began to sink. With his last breath, the frog gasped, "Why did you do that? You fool. Now we both die. Why?"

The scorpion said, "Because it's in my nature." And then they both sank to the bottom of the river.

This timeless tale, shrouded in mystery, fascinates us because its origins are unknown, suggesting that its lessons transcend any single author or culture. The anonymity invites us to reflect on the universal truths it conveys, unbound by specific contexts or narratives.

As we explore various interpretations of the fable, one compelling perspective challenges us to reconsider the notion of innate human nature. This interpretation suggests that many behaviors we perceive as inherent traits are actually learned. For example, our reactions to situations like jealousy are acquired through experiences and social conditioning. This challenges us to question our assumptions about human behavior and the roles of upbringing and environment in shaping it.

However, while acknowledging the influence of learned behaviors, we must also recognize the complexities of human nature. Some behaviors may indeed be learned, but there are undoubtedly innate tendencies that influence our actions. This nuanced understanding allows us to appreciate the interplay between nature and nurture in shaping who we are.

Furthermore, the fable invites us to consider the role of trust in relationships. Some might interpret the story as a cautionary tale against blindly trusting others, but a deeper analysis reveals a more nuanced message. Trust is not simply a binary concept but a dynamic process requiring discernment and understanding. Before placing our trust in others, we must assess their intentions and character, considering their past actions as well as their underlying values and beliefs. Just as the frog should have been wary of the scorpion's nature, we too must be vigilant in evaluating the trustworthiness of those around us.

The fable also prompts us to reflect on responsibility and accountability. While it may be tempting to blame others for betraying our trust, ultimately, we must take ownership of our choices and decisions. This includes recognizing our role in enabling harmful behaviors and learning from these experiences to make wiser choices in the future.

In this sense, the fable serves as a powerful reminder of the importance of self-awareness and discernment in navigating relationships. By understanding the complexities of human nature and exercising prudence in whom we trust, we can cultivate deeper and more meaningful connections with others. Self-awareness is the cornerstone of emotional intelligence, enabling us to recognize our strengths, weaknesses, and motivations. By introspecting and reflecting on our own experiences, we gain insights into our values, fears, and desires. This self-awareness not only allows us to make better decisions for ourselves but also enhances our ability to understand and empathize with others.

In the context of the fable, the frog's lack of self-awareness is evident in its failure to recognize the scorpion's nature. Similarly, in real-life relationships, our blind spots and biases can cloud our judgment, leading us to trust or mistrust others based on faulty assumptions. However, by cultivating self-awareness, we develop a deeper understanding of our own behaviors and reactions. This self-knowledge serves as a valuable lens through which to interpret the actions of others. For instance, if we recognize that we tend to be overly trusting or skeptical, we can approach new relationships with greater caution or openness accordingly.

Understanding our own values and priorities allows us to discern whether others align with them. Just as the frog should have considered whether the scorpion's intentions were compatible with its own survival, we must assess whether the people we choose to trust share our fundamental beliefs and goals. Self-awareness fosters empathy, enabling us to put ourselves in others' shoes and understand their perspectives more deeply. By recognizing our own vulnerabilities and struggles, we become more attuned to the complexities of human nature and more compassionate towards others' shortcomings.

In essence, knowing oneself is not just about introspection; it's about using that self-knowledge as a foundation for understanding and connecting with others. By recognizing our own biases and limitations, we can approach relationships with humility and curiosity, seeking to learn from and about the people we encounter. Ultimately, the journey of self-discovery is ongoing, but it is a journey worth embarking on. By deepening our understanding of ourselves, we enhance our capacity to navigate the complexities of human relationships with wisdom, empathy, and authenticity.

The fable of the scorpion and the frog offers profound insights into human nature, trust, and responsibility. By exploring its various interpretations and implications, we gain a deeper understanding of ourselves and the world around us, empowering us to navigate relationships with wisdom and discernment.

CONFIRMATION BIAS

In the intricate landscape of human cognition, confirmation bias stands as a formidable adversary, quietly shaping our perceptions, decisions, and interactions in ways we often fail to recognize. Its influence is widespread, extending into every aspect of our daily lives and coloring the lens through which we view the world. Understanding confirmation bias is not merely an intellectual exercise; it's a crucial step toward self-awareness and personal growth.

Confirmation bias, at its core, is the tendency to seek, interpret, and remember information in a way that confirms our preexisting beliefs or hypotheses while disregarding or downplaying contradictory evidence. This cognitive bias manifests in various forms and affects virtually every domain of human cognition, from our perceptions of others to our decision-making processes.

Imagine you have a strong belief in the benefits of a particular diet plan. When browsing through articles or social media posts related to nutrition, you are more likely to click on and engage with content that supports your belief in the effectiveness of that diet while ignoring or dismissing articles that present conflicting evidence.

Suppose you hold a negative perception of a coworker based on a few past interactions. In subsequent encounters, you interpret their actions and words in a way that reinforces your initial impression, attributing negative motives to their behavior even when it may be harmless.

You attend a political rally where the speaker presents compelling arguments in support of a certain policy. Later, when discussing the rally with friends, you vividly recall the points that align with your political views while forgetting or distorting information that contradicts your beliefs.

Confirmation bias can have profound implications for our personal and professional lives, influencing the way we form opinions, make decisions, and interact with others. By selectively filtering information, we create echo chambers that reinforce our existing beliefs, narrowing our perspectives and hindering our ability to consider alternative viewpoints. Understanding the psychological mechanisms underlying confirmation bias can shed light on why we are susceptible to its influence.

Several factors contribute to our tendency to seek out confirming evidence and disregard conflicting information:

- **Cognitive Ease:** Processing information that aligns with our beliefs requires less cognitive effort than critically evaluating opposing viewpoints. As a result, we are inclined to gravitate toward information that feels familiar and comfortable, even if it lacks objectivity.

- **Emotional Investment:** Our beliefs are often intertwined with our sense of identity and self-worth. Admitting that we may be wrong challenges not only our intellectual integrity but also our emotional well-being. As a result, we are motivated to defend our beliefs and resist information that threatens them.

- **Social Influence:** Human beings are inherently social creatures, and our beliefs are often shaped by the patterns and values of our social groups. Conforming to the opinions of our peers can provide a sense of belonging and acceptance, incentivizing us to seek out information that aligns with group consensus.

Confirmation bias manifests in various contexts of daily life, illustrating its pervasive influence and the challenges it poses to objective reasoning:

Consider a couple who have been together for several years. When conflicts arise, each person may interpret the other's actions in a way that confirms what they already believe about the relationship. So, if one partner believes their significant other is inconsiderate, they'll only notice the times their partner forgets to do something thoughtful, ignoring all the times they do.

In the workplace, confirmation bias can impact decision-making processes, leading to suboptimal outcomes. A manager tasked with evaluating job candidates may unconsciously favor applicants who fit their preconceived notions of an ideal candidate, overlooking qualifications or experience that challenge their assumptions.

In the world of politics, confirmation bias is like the fuel that keeps the fire burning. People tend to surround themselves with news and opinions that align with their own beliefs, reinforcing their views and making it harder to see things from another perspective.

Luckily, there are ways to outsmart confirmation bias and see the world more clearly:

1. **Mix It Up**

    Expose yourself to different ideas and perspectives. Seek out information that challenges your beliefs rather than just sticking to what you already know. It's like trying new foods—you might discover something you love!

2. **Check Yourself**

    Be aware of your own biases and question your assumptions. Ask yourself, "Am I only paying attention to information that confirms what I believe? Could there be another way to look at this?"

3. **Take a Time-Out**

When you come across information that contradicts your beliefs, don't dismiss it right away. Take a step back, breathe, and give it some thought. Maybe there's something valuable in there that you hadn't considered before.

4. **Stay Curious**

    Approach life with a sense of curiosity and openness. Be willing to change your mind if new evidence comes to light. Remember, it's okay to not have all the answers!

5. **Embrace Cognitive Dissonance**

    Cognitive dissonance occurs when we hold conflicting beliefs or ideas. Instead of avoiding this discomfort, embrace it as an opportunity for growth. Explore the tension between your beliefs and be open to adjusting them in light of new information.

6. **Seek Feedback**

    Regularly seek feedback from others, especially those with different perspectives. Constructive criticism can help you identify blind spots and challenge your assumptions, leading to personal and intellectual growth.

Confirmation bias may be a tricky adversary, but armed with awareness and a willingness to challenge our own thinking, we can overcome its influence. By seeking out diverse perspectives, questioning our assumptions, and staying open to new ideas, we can navigate the twists and turns of our minds with greater clarity and wisdom. So, let's embrace the challenge, break free from the confines of bias, and embark on a journey of discovery—one open-minded step at a time!

NAIVE OPTIMISM

In the pile of life's challenges, one often finds solace in the warmth of optimism. Yet, there exists a particular breed of optimism that dances on the edge of innocence and wisdom - Naive Optimism. It's the unfettered belief that amidst the storms of life, there's a silver lining waiting to be discovered.

Before delving into its benefits, it's essential to comprehend what naive optimism truly entails. Naive optimism isn't about being blind to reality; rather, it's about viewing challenges through a lens of possibility and resilience. It's the audacious belief that every setback is merely a setup for a comeback. Naive optimists possess an unwavering faith in the inherent goodness of life, trusting that even in the darkest of nights, dawn awaits.

Consider the journey of aspiring professional athletes. From the crack of dawn to the setting sun, they devote countless hours honing their craft, facing rejection and setbacks at every turn.

Take the story of Alex, a young football player with dreams of making it to the NFL. Despite the astronomical odds stacked against him (only .2% actually make it), Alex's naive optimism serves as a beacon of hope in his darkest moments. Each missed catch, every defeat on the field, only fuels his determination to defy the odds. While many would falter in the face of such adversity, Alex persists, knowing that every practice session brings him one step closer to his dream.

In the world of professional sports, the path to success is paved with blood, sweat, and tears. Yet, millions of aspiring athletes around the globe continue to chase their dreams with unwavering optimism. They understand the inherent risks and challenges that come with pursuing a career in sports, yet they refuse to be deterred by the naysayers and doubters. It is their naive optimism that propels them forward, pushing them to surpass their limits and achieve greatness against all odds.

As we reflect on the journey of these aspiring athletes, we're reminded of the transformative power of naive optimism. It's not just about believing in the possibility of success; it's about embracing the journey with open arms, knowing that every setback is a stepping stone towards greatness. So, whether you're chasing a career in sports or pursuing your passions in other realms of life, let the story of these resilient athletes serve as a testament to the boundless potential that lies within each of us. With naive optimism as our guiding light, there's no limit to what we can achieve.

Naive optimists possess an innate ability to think outside the box, unbound by the shackles of conventional wisdom. Take the example of Thomas Edison, whose relentless pursuit of the light bulb embodies naive optimism in action. Despite facing thousands of failures, Edison remained undeterred, viewing each experiment not as a setback but as a step closer to success. It was his naive optimism that fueled his creativity, eventually illuminating the world with his invention.

In an age fraught with anxiety and uncertainty, naive optimism serves as a beacon of hope for weary souls. Maintaining a positive outlook can significantly alleviate symptoms of depression and anxiety. By cultivating a mindset of naive optimism, individuals can mitigate the harmful effects of stress, fostering inner peace and tranquility amidst life's chaos.

Naive optimists radiate an infectious energy that draws others towards them like moths to a flame. Their unwavering belief in the goodness of humanity fosters deeper connections and fosters trust. Consider the tale of Emily, whose naive optimism transformed a strained relationship with her estranged father. Instead of harboring resentment, Emily chose to extend an olive branch, believing in the possibility of reconciliation. It was her naive optimism that paved the way for healing, rekindling a bond that had long been dormant.

Hopefully, now you have a better understanding of Naïve Optimism. But how can you apply it to your life? I've already mentioned a bunch of these examples before. It goes to show you how beneficial they really are.

Practice Gratitude: Start each day by acknowledging the blessings in your life, no matter how small. Cultivating an attitude of gratitude lays the foundation for naive optimism to flourish.

Challenge Negative Thoughts: When faced with adversity, refrain from succumbing to defeatist thinking. Instead, challenge negative thoughts and reframe them in a positive light. Remember, every setback is merely a setup for a comeback.

Visualize Success: Take a moment each day to visualize your goals and aspirations as if they've already been achieved. By manifesting your dreams through visualization, you pave the way for their realization.

Surround Yourself with Positivity: Surround yourself with individuals who exude positivity and optimism. Their energy will uplift and inspire you, reinforcing your own naive optimism.

Embrace Failure as Growth: View failure not as a reflection of your abilities but as an opportunity for growth and learning. Embrace setbacks with open arms, knowing that they are integral to the journey towards success.

Naive optimism isn't just a fleeting emotion; it's a way of life—a powerful tool that empowers us to transcend obstacles and embrace the limitless possibilities that lie ahead. By embracing naive optimism, we unlock the door to a world of boundless potential, where every challenge is an opportunity and every setback a stepping stone towards greatness. So, dare to dream, dare to believe, and watch as the universe conspires to make your wildest dreams a reality.

REFLECTIONS ON LIFE'S LESSONS

Life unfolds as a continuous journey of learning and growth, a narrative woven with experiences that shape our understanding and mold our character. From the earliest moments of existence, we are immersed in a classroom without walls, where challenges and opportunities alike present themselves as invaluable teachers. Each encounter, whether joyful or fraught with hardship, contributes to our development and well-being, imparting lessons that resonate throughout our lives.

The Foundations of Learning

In infancy, we embark on the arduous yet exhilarating journey of mastering the art of walking. With unsteady steps and determined hearts, we navigate the terrain of our world, often stumbling and falling along the way. Yet, with each tumble, we glean a profound lesson in resilience and determination. We discover that setbacks are not signs of defeat but rather stepping stones on the path to mastery. Supported by the unwavering encouragement of our loved ones, we learn that perseverance and courage are the bedrock upon which we build our dreams.

Navigating the Flames of Experience

As we mature, we encounter new challenges that test our understanding of risk and consequence. The stove becomes a metaphor for the dual nature of the world—both a source of warmth and sustenance and a potential hazard. Through the searing pain of burns, we gain a visceral understanding of caution and respect, learning to tread carefully amidst life's fiery trials. Yet, in embracing these lessons, we also discover the transformative power of resilience, harnessing adversity to fuel our growth and culinary creativity.

Life's Lessons

Life teaches us through many experiences beyond childhood, shaping our beliefs, values, and dreams. These experiences include both successes and failures. By facing and overcoming failures, we develop resilience and perseverance. This process helps us learn to navigate difficult times with grace and strength. Each challenge we overcome contributes to our growth, making us better equipped to handle future obstacles. In this way, life's lessons extend far beyond our early years, continually molding us into stronger, more capable individuals.

Recalling and Revisiting

Yet, amidst life's myriad distractions and tribulations, it is all too easy to lose sight of the lessons we have learned or to allow self-doubt to cloud our judgment. We may succumb to the siren song of negativity, surrendering our dreams to the dissonance of doubt and fear. Yet, it is in these moments of darkness that the wisdom of our experiences shines most brightly. By heeding the counsel of our past selves, we can navigate life's twists and turns with clarity and purpose, embracing failure as a catalyst for growth and adversity to use it as a springboard for resilience.

The Ever-Evolving Journey

Life's lessons are not static but rather fluid, evolving alongside our experiences and aspirations. To stagnate is to deny ourselves the opportunity for growth and self-discovery. It is upon us to remain vigilant in our pursuit of knowledge and to apply the lessons we have learned to our current circumstances. By doing so, we unlock the boundless potential within us, charting a course toward fulfillment and self-actualization.

Every triumph and tribulation serves as a thread, weaving together the fabric of our lives. As we traverse the labyrinth of experience, let us embrace the wisdom gleaned from our journey, drawing strength from the lessons learned and forging ahead with courage and conviction. For in the crucible of life's challenges, we discover the true essence of our humanity and the boundless potential that lies within.

CONCLUSION

As we reach the conclusion of our journey through **"A Logical Guide to Happiness"** it's essential to reflect on the profound wisdom we've uncovered and the transformative potential it holds for our lives.

Throughout this book, we've delved deep into the intricacies of the human experience, exploring topics ranging from freewill and happiness to mindset and resilience. We've uncovered invaluable insights into the power of self-awareness, gratitude, and perspective, discovering that true fulfillment lies not in the pursuit of external accolades or material possessions, but in the cultivation of inner peace, purpose, and authenticity.

We've learned that life is a journey filled with both triumphs and tribulations, and that our response to adversity ultimately shapes our character and defines our destiny. By embracing challenges with courage, resilience, and an unwavering belief in our own potential, we can transform obstacles into opportunities and emerge stronger, wiser, and more resilient than ever before.

As we've explored the power of mindset and attitude, we've come to understand that our thoughts and beliefs have a profound impact on our experiences and perceptions of the world. By adopting a growth mindset, cultivating gratitude, and reframing challenges as opportunities for growth and learning, we can navigate life's twists and turns with greater ease and grace, finding meaning and fulfillment in even the most difficult of circumstances.

But perhaps most importantly, we've discovered the transformative potential of each and every one of us. That we have the power to pave our own path. That our own happiness and well-being is within our power to obtain. That with effort and an open mind all that we wish for is a possibility.

As we bid farewell to these pages, let us carry forth the lessons we've learned and the insights we've gained into our daily lives. Let us approach each day with courage, curiosity, and an unwavering belief in the power of the human spirit to overcome adversity and create a brighter, more compassionate world for ourselves and future generations.

May the wisdom contained within these pages serve as a guiding light on your journey through life, illuminating the path forward and empowering you to navigate life's challenges with grace, resilience, and an unwavering belief in the boundless potential that lies within each of us.

Thank you for joining us on this transformative journey. May your path be filled with love, joy, and abundance, and may you continue to grow and evolve into the best possible version of yourself.

ACKNOWLEDGEMENTS

First and foremost, I want to express that writing this has been a labor of love. The journey took several years and was often challenging and frustrating, yet profoundly rewarding.

I want to emphasize this:

If I can do it, so can any of you.

With that being said, there are several people to whom I owe a great deal of gratitude for helping me through this process, whether through direct assistance, inspiration, or unwavering support.

To my parents, Nino and Mary: your unwavering support for all my wild ideas has been my foundation. Thank you for always believing in me.

To my sisters, Nicole and Elizabeth, and my brother-in-law, Francesco: your constant encouragement and ability to keep me grounded while making me believe that anything is possible have been invaluable.

To my nephews, Cristian and Daniel: your presence inspires me every day to be the best role model I can be.

To my friends, Cosimo, Rocco, Sam, Nancy, Mirella, Daniella, Nancy, and Daniel (and any others I may have inadvertently left out): thank you for your insightful conversations, debates, and unwavering belief in my abilities. Your companionship and support have been crucial.

To those who have crossed my path and inspired me in one way or another—Rossana, Roza, Shirley, Lisa, Simone, and any others whose names I may have forgotten—your influence has been deeply felt.

I am profoundly grateful to all of you. Your support, encouragement, and belief in me have made this journey possible. Thank you from the bottom of my heart.

www.ingramcontent.com/pod-product-compliance
Lightning Source LLC
Chambersburg PA
CBHW051559010526
44118CB00023B/2750